THE KILLER'S HENCHMAN

BOOKS BY STEPHEN GOWANS

Washington's Long War on Syria (2017)

Patriots, Traitors and Empires: The Story of Korea's Struggle for Freedom (2018)

Israel, A Beachhead in the Middle East: From European Colony to US Power Projection Platform

THE KILLER'S HENCHMAN

Capitalism and the Covid-19 Disaster

By Stephen Gowans

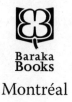

Baraka
Books

Montréal

© Baraka Books

ISBN 978-1-77186-274-5 pbk; 978-1-77186-284-4 epub; 978-1-77186-285-1 pdf

Cover by Maison 1608
Book Design by Folio infographie
Editing and proofreading: Robin Philpot, Anne Marie Marko, Amelia Delli Quadri

Legal Deposit, 2nd quarter 2022
Bibliothèque et Archives nationales du Québec
Library and Archives Canada

Published by Baraka Books of Montreal

Printed and bound in Quebec

Trade Distribution & Returns
Canada – UTP Distribution: UTPdistribution.com

United States
Independent Publishers Group: IPGbook.com

We acknowledge the support from the Société de développement des entreprises culturelles (SODEC) and the Government of Quebec tax credit for book publishing administered by SODEC.

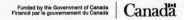

CONTENTS

And here it becomes evident that the bourgeoisie is unfit any longer to be the ruling class in society. — Karl Marx

PREFACE

*Accumulation of wealth at one pole is, therefore,
at the same time, accumulation of misery, agony of toil,
slavery, ignorance, brutality, mental degradation
at the opposite pole.* — Friedrich Engels[1]

In the summer of 2021, as the novel coronavirus scythed through populations around the world, the World Health Organization's director-general, Tedros Adhanom Ghebreyesus announced that the pandemic will end "when the world chooses to end it."[2] "We have all the tools we need," Tedros said. "Proven public health and social measures; rapid and accurate diagnostics; effective therapeutics including oxygen; and of course, powerful vaccines."[3]

And yet the pandemic didn't end.

The proven health and social measures Tedros mentioned—that China, South Korea, New Zealand, and a handful of other countries had used to drive infections to zero—were shunned by much of the rest of the world, in favor of allowing the virus to run riot, or imposing half measures, and only when hospitals were under an unbearable strain.

If public health and social measures were eschewed, vaccines were embraced. They were promoted as a cavalry that would rescue humanity from the virus. But when the cavalry arrived, it found itself unable to vanquish the enemy. Countries that rolled out vaccines quickly to the willing parts of their populations, soon turned to boosters in a vain attempt to push back the unrelentingly advancing virus.

Meanwhile, a global vaccine apartheid left poor- and middle-income countries at the back of the queue, waiting for crumbs to fall from the rich countries' table, as new, possibly more virulent variants, threatened to emerge from an accelerating viral vortex.

While much of the world suffered owing to the failure of governments to use the tools available to them, a small minority thrived.

Major figures in the pharmaceutical industry became billionaires, as their companies' share prices soared in response to the "vaccine strategy" embraced by the United States and its satellites—an approach to the pandemic adopted by governments based on an idea, vigorously promoted by the billionaire Bill Gates, that vaccines, manufactured by the private sector with public sector support, could be the main weapon in the fight against Covid-19. Drug and biotech companies, including Moderna, Pfizer, BioNTech, and AstraZeneca, received substantial injections of public sector funding, support, and technology, to supply much of the world with immunizations against the advancing virus. The companies' major shareholders—including key members of the Trump and Biden administrations—were soon awash in riches.

The collective worth of the planet's 2,690 billionaires grew by over $8 trillion, from a pre-pandemic $5 trillion to $13.5 trillion by the summer of 2021. Jeff Bezos' wealth alone grew by over $79 billion, accumulated out of the labor of poorly paid and highly exploited Amazon workers.[4] Bezos' pandemic gains were enough to give each of his 876,000 employees a $91,000 pandemic bonus. He declined. Instead, 4,000 Amazon workers in nine US states signed up for food stamps to get by on Bezos' paltry payouts.[5]

So it was that as the dark shadow of Covid-19 descended upon workers and the poor, it smiled beatifically upon the billionaire class. Jamie Dimon, chief executive officer of JPMorgan Chase & Co—a plutocrat whose influence reaches deep into the White House—could boast that "our cup runneth over."[6] *The Wall Street*

Journal noted that the pandemic left Corporate USA flushed with cash, "ready to pad shareholder pockets."[7]

The pain of the world's majority, and the gain of the infinitesimal billionaire minority, was the outcome of the latter having long used its vast wealth to buy political influence over the former, and to shape government responses to the pandemic to its own agenda, not humanity's.

The billionaire class, imperiously guided by capitalist imperatives, shaped the response to the viral crisis in four ways: First, it eschewed the public health and social measures that China showed could be used successfully to eliminate infections and that the WHO endorsed, believing a robust public health approach would interfere with profit-making and hurt the stock market. Instead, and second, it promoted vaccines as the main way out of the pandemic, funneling untold billions of dollars of public sector funding to itself and the biopharmaceutical firms it controlled. Third, it placed the burden of mitigating the pandemic on small business owners, whose businesses were shuttered, allowing Amazon to fill the void and expand significantly. Fourth, it plunged "essential" workers—in reality "sacrificial" workers—into the dark abyss of Covid-19, providing insufficient protection on the job, and inadequate financial support to self-isolate when ill.

Capitalism, its incentives, its power to dominate the political process, and its elevation of profit-making above all other considerations, prevented humanity from using the tools Tedros identified as sufficient to end the pandemic. The result was over five million confirmed deaths worldwide two years into the pandemic, and many more due to unrelated illness or injury that could not be treated owing to pandemic pressure on medical resources.

Could an alternative system have done better? China, while not a break with capitalist economics—the country has a thriving capitalism and a growing number of billionaires—is sufficiently different from the capitalism of much of the rest of the world to discern what might have happened in a world where capitalist imperatives are not wholly in command. It is not billionaires pursuing profit-making goals that rule the East Asian colossus, but Communists pursuing the public policy goals of economic development and national rejuvenation. State-owned enterprises guided by five-year plans lie at the center of the Chinese economy, and the state has investments in innumerable private firms, allowing Beijing to guide China's economic life along lines that comport with Communist goals.

China's pandemic performance was without equal—a public health marvel that richly deserved the praise the West refused to grant. By means of non-pharmaceutical public health measures, the country rapidly eliminated community transmission of the virus, allowing its economy to reopen quickly and safely. At the same time, it developed its own vaccines, and inoculated most of its people. Two years into the pandemic, the number of US Americans that had died in an average week was greater than the total number of Chinese that had died over more than 100 weeks. Had the world emulated China's epidemic control measures, there would have been no pandemic; no protracted serial lockdowns; no prolonged disruption to people's livelihoods; and no viral Golgotha.

But the United States is not so different from China that we can't also discern in the US model whether a different system could have done better. Like China—and contrary to the mythology of US free enterprise—the US economy pivots on the public sector. The technology behind the Moderna and Pfizer-BioNTech vaccines was developed in publicly-funded university and government labs, as have so many other innovations, from the Internet to most of the components of the iPhone. These innovations, produced at public expense, were transferred to private hands, for private gain. BioNTech licensed from the US government and the University of Pennsylvania the technology behind the vaccine it produced with Pfizer, while Moderna licensed University of Pennsylvania research and additionally collaborated on its vaccine with the US government's National Institutes of Health.[8] US government scientists call Moderna's shot the NIH-Moderna vaccine, with the NIH given precedence to reflect the primacy of the government's role. In the US orbit, Covid-19 vaccines wouldn't have been possible without the logistical support of the Pentagon, and billions of dollars in publicly-funded research and advance purchase agreements from Washington and other governments.

The Pentagon's logistical expertise could have been used to run a mass testing and contact tracing program *à la* Chinese, along with the building and management of quarantine facilities, with the reward of the better part of a million lives saved. Tens of billions of dollars could have been spent on providing financial support to infected workers, so they could have taken time off the job to quarantine. Vaccines and therapeutics could have been produced by state-owned companies, cutting out private investors, whose only contribution to drug development was to charge grossly inflated prices for treatments developed by the public sector, and then to collect a dividend as the culmination of their parasitism.

The US model is socialist, no matter how much government officials and their billionaire patrons would like us to think otherwise. But it's a socialism for the rich. It's time to replace this faux socialism with socialism as it is intended to be—under democratic control; unfettered by profit-making imperatives that prevent us from using all the tools at our disposal for the solution of common problems; and free to realize the promise inherent in science, technology, and industry of a world free from unnecessary toil, disease, ignorance, poverty, and environmental degradation.

To be sure, it sounds utopian. But consider this: By the close of 2021, more than two full years after a novel coronavirus had jumped the species barrier to humans, only 4,636 people had died from the virus in China, a country of 1.4 billion people. Had fatalities accumulated at the same rate as in the United States, nearly 3.5 million Chinese would have perished. Looked at another way, China was able to realize the potential of basic, widely-known, and long-established non-pharmaceutical epidemic control measures to save millions of lives, because capitalist imperatives weren't in charge and Communists animated by public welfare goals were. In proportion as capitalist imperatives are weakened, what people are able to accomplish collectively is vastly expanded.

In the early 1940s, US folk singer Woody Guthrie sang of *A Better World A Coming*. Guthrie's better world rested on a vision of a socialist future. A better world is coming, but it's one we'll have to make together. The first step, as two German philosophers wrote in 1848, is to replace the rule of billionaires—that is, to win the battle for democracy.

CHAPTER 1

THE KILLER

"Covid is a highly transmissible infection; it's substantially novel to human immune systems and provokes severe symptoms in some cases; with enough cases hitting at the same time, hospital systems are likely to be overwhelmed in direct measure to their pre-existing capacity or lack thereof." – Holman W. Jenkins Jr.[1]

"In any previous war, the US did not lose over 4,400 people in one day." – Hu Xijin[2]

The emergence of new pathogens—viruses, bacteria, and other disease-causing organisms—is inevitable. But pandemics—outbreaks of illness on a global scale leading to overwhelmed healthcare systems and major economic upheaval—are optional. SARS-CoV-2, the virus that causes Covid-19, created a global disaster. But, as the World Health Organization's Independent Experts' Panel pointed out, the disaster was preventable. It didn't have to happen.[3]

There are five types of pathogens: viruses, bacteria, funguses, protozoa, and parasitic worms. Viruses are bits of genetic material encased in a protein shell. They hijack cells to produce copies of themselves and in the process, damage or kill the cells they invade. Influenza, or the flu (along with Covid-19), is caused by viruses.

Bacteria are single cell organisms that cause illness by producing toxins. Tuberculosis, cholera, tetanus, Lyme disease, and some sexually transmitted afflictions, are caused by bacteria. Protozoa are single cell organisms that move through water and parasitize their host. Malaria, a disease of periodic chills and fever, enlargement of the spleen, and anemia, is caused by a protozoan transmitted by mosquitoes. Funguses are responsible for such diseases as Athlete's foot and ringworm. They are single- or multi-cell organisms that are able to survive outside a host.

Occasionally new pathogens are transmitted to humans from other vertebrate animals. These cause zoonoses, from the Greek, *zoo* (animal) and *nosos* (disease). According to the World Health Organization (WHO), zoonoses:

- Can spread to humans through direct contact or indirectly through food, water, or the environment.
- May be bacterial, viral, or parasitic.
- Comprise a large percentage of new and existing diseases in humans.

There are many zoonoses. Covid-19 is one of them.

New pathogens are dangerous because we have no immunological defense against them. They can spread easily and rapidly from one person to another, until a large number of people fall ill at the same time. A sudden rapid increase in illness can have devastating consequences for healthcare systems and economies, especially in poor countries where healthcare may be inadequate, or in countries weakened by economic sanctions (which are almost invariably low- and middle-income) and whose governments may already struggle to meet their populations' healthcare and nutritional needs. Even if a novel pathogen causes mild or moderate illness for most people, as is true of SARS-Cov-2, it is still possible that the pathogen could cause serious illness in enough people that hospitals are overwhelmed and employee absenteeism skyrockets, creating major economic upheaval.

Here's what would have happened had measures not been taken to control the spread of the novel coronavirus, according to UCLA economist Andrew Atkeson:[4]

- Plotting the course of the virus's spread by day, in fairly quick order, the number of people infected would climb to 10 percent of the population. One in 10 workers would be off the job.
- Another set of workers would take time off to care for sick children and relatives.
- While most infected people would recover at home with mild to moderate illness, the number of people requiring medical attention would exceed hospital capacity. In high-income countries, hospitals can accommodate 0.40 percent of the population at any given time, under normal circumstances.[5] Approximately seven percent of Covid-19 patients require hospitalization.[6] With one in 10 infected at the pandemic's peak, (1/10 x 7 percent=) 0.70 percent would need to be hospitalized. The number exceeds hospital capacity by close to a factor of two.
- One in 10 doctors and nurses, and possibly more, would fall ill. One in 10 non-medical staff would also be sick. Healthcare worker absenteeism would reduce the capacity of already strained hospitals to care for those requiring urgent medical attention.
- The corpses of those who succumbed to the infection would pile up in refrigerator trucks and temporary morgues. The corpses of others who required urgent medical attention for other illnesses and injuries, but were turned away from overwhelmed hospitals, would add to the expanding Golgotha.
- Terrified by the collapse of the healthcare system, and the ubiquity of temporary morgues, people would self-isolate. Absenteeism would soar.
- Rising employee absenteeism would paralyze the economy.

In a pandemic, the infected either die, or survive and develop some form of immunity. The more people who acquire immunity, the fewer pathways the pathogen can follow to infect the people who aren't immune. Eventually, the populace reaches population immunity (often called "herd immunity" and sometimes "community protection")—the point at which the rate of the pathogen's spread begins to decelerate as the number of immunologically naïve hosts dwindles. The number of infections drops to a low level, manageable by hospital and other healthcare resources.

The World Health Organization and many scientists believe that the emergence of new pathogens, particularly those which come from other animals, is inevitable, and that pandemics are becoming highly likely. This represents a radical shift in thinking from the mid-twentieth century, when it was widely believed that we were undergoing an epidemiological transition—a major shift in the kinds of diseases we would face in the future.

By 1948, the development of vaccines and antibiotics, in conjunction with public health measures to control the spread of infectious disease, led doctors and scientists to believe that humanity was poised on the cusp of a new era in human history. It appeared that the scourge of infectious disease, which had plagued humanity for millennia, would become, if not eradicated, then virtually eliminated. The Nobel Prize-winning virologist Frank Macfarlane Burnet declared in 1962 that, "To write about infectious diseases is almost to write of something that has passed into history."[7] He conceded that a "totally unexpected" outbreak might occur, but that "the most likely forecast about the future of infectious disease is that it will be very dull."[8] Seven years later, an effusive US "Surgeon General declared an end to infectious diseases. Public health agencies predicted that the infectious maladies that had afflicted humanity for centuries, from malaria to smallpox, would be eradicated by the end of the twentieth century. Responding to this grand optimism, schools of medicine closed their departments of infectious diseases."[9]

The optimism proved groundless. Five decades later, only one infectious disease has yielded to human intervention: small pox. Rather than disappearing, infectious disease as a class has expanded as new contagions surface. Between 1980 and 2006, 335 new microbial threats were identified, most of them of zoonotic origin.[10] Since 1960, three quarters of new infectious diseases have been zoonoses.[11] And since 2002, the world has been menaced in varying degrees by six new zoonotic afflictions: three corona-viruses (SARS, Middle East Respiratory Syndrome or MERS, and Covid-19); Ebola; Zika; and Nipah. In the last decade, the World Health Organization has declared a "public-health emergency of international concern" in connection with six infectious diseases: the H1N1 influenza, swine flu, polio, Ebola, Zika, and Covid-19.[12]

To be sure, the emergence of over three hundred new infectious maladies since 1980 may be less a sign of a growing biological threat and more an indication of scientific advance in the identification of pathogens. Moreover, not all new pathogens are threats to human-ity and most are limited in time and space, confined geographically and infecting few. Notably, while SARS, MERS, Ebola, swine flu, Zika, and Nipah have caused problems and killed many, they have not disrupted healthcare systems and economies on a world scale.

***

The Great Influenza pandemic of 1918 to 1920 is a model of a novel infection with seismic consequences. Known colloquially as the Spanish Flu, the influenza was caused by the H1N1 virus. The virus originated in birds, passing to humans possibly in China, France, or the United States. One hundred years later, the virus's origins remain murky. The zoonotic pathogen infected 620 mil-lion people, about one out of every three people alive at the time. Over 40 million fell ill with the disease in the United States, and two million were sickened in Canada. The sudden, rapid onset of illness engulfing a substantial proportion of the world's population, severely disrupted economic activity, and plunged the global econ-omy into crisis. Economically, the Great Influenza pandemic was the fourth greatest global calamity of the twentieth century, after World War II, the Great Depression, and World War I.

The virus was also possibly the greatest cause of death from a pathogen over a limited number of years in human history. It killed 50 million to 100 million people worldwide, about 2.5 to five percent of the world's population, equivalent to 212 million to 424 million people today. The enormity of the disaster can best be understood if we consider that were a pandemic of this scale to strike today, it would wipe out a population equivalent to that of the United States. Close to 750,000 people died in North America. Most of the world's fatalities—from 60 percent to two-thirds—occurred in Western India, where a famine, induced by a British decision to divert grain to troops in Europe, left the Indian population weakened, malnourished, and ill-equipped to fight off disease.[13]

War and pandemics have often been compared. In his 1947 novel, *The Plague*, Albert Camus noted that: "Everybody knows that pestilences have a way of recurring in the world; yet somehow we find it hard to believe in ones that crash down on our heads from a blue sky. There have been as many plagues as wars in history; yet always plagues and wars take people equally by surprise." Ironically, while wars are often remembered and dreaded for their carnage, plagues are often forgotten and their consequence underestimated. In their textbook, *Infectious Diseases of Humans*, Roy M. Anderson and Robert M. May noted that "A catalogue of the number of deaths induced by major epidemics of historical times is staggering, and dwarfs the total deaths on all past battlefields."[14] The preponderance of death due to infectious disease over death due to war was no less true in the twentieth century.[15] The number of influenza deaths worldwide from 1918-1920 alone surpassed the number of fatalities in World War I (17 million), World War II (60 million), and possibly both wars combined. Moreover, at some points during the Covid-19 pandemic, more US citizens were "dying of the coronavirus every month, on average, than died in the deadliest month of World War II."[16]

Five great wars in US history produced major US fatalities. The deadliest was the Civil War, which claimed 620,000 lives, more US Americans than perished in World War I, World War II, the Korean

War, or the Vietnam War. In absolute number of deaths, the Covid-19 pandemic was more deadly in the United States than all of the five great wars, including the Civil War. As many US Americans died from Covid-19 by January 22, 2021 as died in World War II (418,500) and as many perished to August 12, 2021 as were whisked away by the hand of death in the Civil War.

But comparing absolute numbers presents a problem. The longer a death event lasts, the greater the opportunity for fatalities to accumulate. In order to compare like to like, we need to place fatalities on a common scale. One way to do this is to look at the average number of deaths per day over the course of a death event.

When death events are examined this way, the Covid-19 pandemic reveals itself to be more deadly than all the great wars. Over 1,150 US citizens died daily, on average, from 19 January 2020, the day the first Covid-19 case was confirmed in the United States, to 31 December 2021. The deadliest war, the Civil War, at 427 deaths per day on average, is a distant second.

Yet, no matter how deadly the Covid-19 pandemic, there was one more deadly: the influenza pandemic of 1918-1920. That pandemic killed an estimated 675,000 US citizens, or 1,232 per day on average, slightly more than the daily number killed by the novel coronavirus.

However, the comparison is partly misleading. The US population was much smaller when the Great Influenza struck. Adjusting for population growth, the flu pandemic was more deadly. Looking

US deaths caused by Covid-19 vs. US deaths in war

	Deaths	Days	Deaths per day. avg.
Covid-19*	824,240	712	1,158
Civil War	620,000	1,451	427
World War II	418,500	1,365	307
World War I	116,516	591	197
Korean War	36,516	1,127	32
Vietnam War	58,209	4,380	13

*January 19, '20 – December 31, '21

US deaths caused by pandemics

	Deaths	Days	Deaths per day. avg.
Influenza pandemic 1918-1920	675,000	548	1,232
Covid-19*	824,240	712	1,158

*January 19, '20 – December 31, '21

at fatalities per million, the Civil War was by far the deadliest event in US history, both in the cumulative number of deaths and the average number of deaths per day. The influenza pandemic of 1918-1920 comes second, while the Covid-19 pandemic places a distant third. The coronavirus pestilence and the twentieth century wars comprise a class of their own, much less deadly than the Civil War and the 1918-1920 influenza. Even so, compared to the wars of the last century, the Covid-19 pandemic has been more deadly, even taking population growth into account.

What these findings reveal is that the 1918-1920 Great Influenza and Covid-19 pandemic were major death events in which more US citizens perished than in any of the four major twentieth century wars, controlling for the number of days the death event lasted, along with population size.

US deaths caused by pandemics and wars

	Deaths per million	Days	Deaths per day per million, avg.
Civil War	19,726	1,451	13.6
Influenza pandemic 1918-1920	6,541	548	11.9
Covid-19*	2,480	712	3.5
World War II	3,137	1,365	2.3
World War I	1,128	591	1.9
Korean War	240	1,127	0.2
Vietnam War	303	4,380	0.1

*January 19, '20 – December 31, '21

The Great Influenza was dubbed the Spanish Flu because Spain, neutral during the Great War, was the only country that openly acknowledged the outbreak. Other countries kept their epidemics secret, to avoid publicly disclosing information their enemies might use against them. Since governments other than Spain's were loath to admit they had a problem, they were happy to conceal their own outbreaks behind a name that localized the malady to Spain. While no one knows for sure where the outbreak originated, scientists regard the United States as a leading candidate. Were the unhappy practice of naming pandemics after their presumed country of origin to continue, the influenza of 1918-1920 might be called the US Flu. Another practice was to name the pestilence after an enemy country. The Germans called the influenza the Russian Pest. The Russians called it the Chinese Fever. This convention continued with the Trump administration's efforts to blame China for the Covid-19 pandemic by calling the disease the Wuhan Flu, the Kung Flu, and the China Virus. The Biden administration continued the practice more subtly in efforts to pin the blame for the pandemic on a purported accidental leak from a Wuhan virology laboratory.

The WHO predicts that because population density is growing and people can move quickly about the globe, if a comparably lethal and transmissible contagion jumped the species barrier to humans today, the impact would be even more devastating than it was in 1918. "In addition to tragic levels of mortality, such a pandemic could cause panic, destabilize national security and seriously impact the global economy and trade."[17]

Over the nearly two years the Great Influenza swept hundreds of millions into early graves, enough people acquired immunity through infection that the pandemic—which we can define as a period of major disruption to healthcare systems and the economy as a substantial part of the population falls ill—gradually came to an end. But the H1N1 virus that caused the mayhem never went away. It continued to circulate, passing from humans to animals and back to humans, mutating along the way. The descendants of the original virus remain with us today, as the cause of the seasonal flu, and occasionally as the cause of larger, worldwide outbreaks, as happened in 1957, 1968, and 2009.

Warnings have been repeatedly sounded that a major pathogenic outbreak on the scale of the Great Influenza is on the horizon. In 2012, the Pentagon's policy think tank, the Rand Corporation, pointed to the possibility of a major pandemic engulfing the world. It defined a microbial epidemic as the only threat that poses an existential danger to the United States[18] (notable, given the routine practice of the White House, the Pentagon, and the Western media of presenting such countries as China, Russia, North Korea, and Iran, as existential menaces). The Johns Hopkins Center for Health Security warned in 2018 and 2019 that a novel coronavirus could produce tens of millions of deaths.[19] For its part, the US intelligence community has warned every year from 2013 to 2019 that "History is replete with examples of pathogens sweeping populations that lack immunity, causing political and economic upheaval."[20] On the eve of the Covid-19 pandemic, a Chinese scientist predicted the emergence of a "future SARS- or MERS-like coronavirus," likely in China, originating in bats. His prediction was based on research that found that people living in rural communities in southern China, where there are large bat populations, were being exposed to coronaviruses.[21]

In September 2019, a few months before the first case of Covid-19 was identified, the WHO released a premonitory report titled *A World at Risk*. Noting that the accelerating increase in new infectious diseases was a harbinger of "a new era of high-impact, potentially fast-spreading outbreaks that are more frequently detected and increasingly difficult to manage," the world health body presaged a looming global health emergency. There is, WHO scientists cautioned, "a very real threat of a rapidly moving, highly lethal pandemic of a respiratory pathogen killing 50 to 80 million people and wiping out nearly five percent of the world's economy." A pandemic on this scale, the report noted, "would be catastrophic" and would create "widespread havoc, instability and insecurity." The WHO worried that the world was unprepared.

Presciently, the UN body sketched out the impact of a respiratory pandemic, unaware that the embryonic Covid-19 pandemic lay gestating in its womb. "The great majority of national health systems would be unable to handle a large influx of patients infected with a respiratory pathogen capable of easy transmissibility and high mortality," the report warned. Healthcare systems would be overwhelmed, "reducing access to health services for all diseases and conditions." This would engender "even greater mortality." There would be economic effects, too. "In addition to tragic levels of mortality, such a pandemic could cause panic, destabilize national security and seriously impact the global economy and trade," the report warned.

While many scientists describe pandemics as *inevitable*, it's more accurate to say that if the future resembles the past, pandemics are *highly likely*. Pandemics have occurred repeatedly throughout history, and, despite unduly sanguine mid-twentieth century prognostications about the demise of infectious diseases, pandemics refuse to obligingly withdraw from the stage of human history. History records numerous plagues, cholera pandemics, five flu pandemics since 1918, the AIDS pandemic, and the Covid-19 pandemic. What's more, some of the risk factors that make pandemics more likely are present today to a greater degree than they ever have been.

There are three great risk factors that elevate the likelihood of future pandemics: population growth; increasing population density; and growing interconnectedness among countries and communities.

Population growth increases the risk of a novel disease outbreak for one simple reason: The more people there are, the greater the chance that a novel pathogen will spill over to one of us from another animal species. Since China is the world's most populous country, a zoonotic spillover is more likely to happen there than anywhere else, other things being equal. In population size, India is second to China, and the United States third. Together, these countries account for 40 percent of the world's population, and there is therefore a 40 percent *a priori* chance that if a contagion jumps the species barrier that patient zero will either be Chinese, Indian, or a US American.

As the world's population has grown, humans have crammed tighter together into the earth's finite space. World population density has tripled in the past seven decades, increasing from 18.9 people per square kilometer in 1950 to 58.3 in 2021.[22] By itself, more people in a finite space means a greater chance that if a new pathogen jumps the species barrier to humans, it will find pathways to spread.

The growth of megacities, some teeming with massive slums, makes pathogen transmission all the more likely. Tokyo's population is equal to that of Canada, but the city's footprint is over four thousand times smaller than Canada's. Large populations living in tiny spaces create the perfect conditions for the rapid spread of dangerous microbes. A number of cities have populations larger than many countries. Delhi has over 31 million residents (larger than Venezuela); Shanghai has over 27 million (more populous than all of Australia); Sao Paulo has over 22 million (a greater population than Chile's); while Mexico City has over 21 million (greater than Guatemala). Wuhan, the city in China where Covid-19 was first identified, has over 11 million people (more than live in Sweden). China has 93 cities with populations of one million or more.[23]

Existing societal factors are congenial to the spread of pulmonary infectious disease, observed Frank M. Snowden, an historian of medicine at Yale University. "These include whatever circumstances cause large numbers of people to assemble in crowded spaces, such as urbanization, congested housing, crowded workplaces, and warfare."[24] The industrial revolution created the perfect conditions for the spread of infectious diseases, including mass migration of displaced peasant population to cities, where workers lived in crowded, unhygienic slums, and worked side by side in "dark satanic mills," as the poet William Blake called them.

Many megalopolises teem with favelas, recalling the nineteenth century English working class slums chronicled by Friedrich Engels.

The streets are generally unpaved, rough, dirty, filled with vegetable and animal refuse, without sewers or gutters, but supplied with foul, stagnant pools instead. Moreover, ventilation is impeded by the bad, confused method of building the whole quarter, and since many human beings live crowded into a small space, the atmosphere that prevails in these working-men's quarters may be readily imagined.[25]

Describing the working-class London slum of St. Giles, Engels wrote:

It is a disorderly collection of tall, three or four-storied houses, with narrow, crooked, filthy streets, in which there is quite as much life as in the great thoroughfares of the town, except that, here, people of the working class only are to be seen. A vegetable market is held in the street, baskets with vegetables and fruits, naturally all bad and hardly fit to use, obstruct the sidewalk still further, and from these, as well as from the fish dealers' stalls, arises a horrible smell. The houses are occupied from cellar to garret, filthy within and without, and their appearance is such as no human being could possibly wish to live in them. But all this is nothing compared with the dwellings in the narrow courts and alleys between the streets, entered by covered passages between the houses, in which the filth and tottering ruin surpass all description. ... Heaps of garbage and ashes lie in all directions, and the foul liquids emptied before the doors gather in stinking pools.[26]

Sadly, people continue to live in filthy, overcrowded, unsanitary, stinking shantytowns, in such places as Cape Town, Nairobi, Mumbai, and Karachi. Slum dwellers comprise 900 million people, one quarter of the world's urban population. Their living conditions are petri dishes for pathogens.

The third great pandemic risk factor is the growing number of connections among communities and countries. For much of human history, people lived in small hunting and gathering tribes of no more than one hundred people. Most human interaction occurred within tribes, and little interaction, if any, occurred between them. The tribes were like countries with closed borders. If, say, through contact with bats, a tribe member became infected by a novel coronavirus, the virus might reach a "pandemic" level within the tribe itself but never pass to another. The illness would be confined to the tribe, since, owing to its limited interactions with other communities, chances are the virus would fail to find a human transmission belt into another community. The risk of the pathogen triggering a true pandemic—one in which the virus became almost universally present in all human communities very quickly—would be effectively zero.

As humans began to settle in larger communities, even cities, and to develop trade and exchange with other communities, opportunities for the spread of infectious diseases grew. Still, for much of human history, most people never ventured very far from the region in which they were born. All that has changed. Today, people can—and do—travel by air across vast distances in only a few hours. Most cities in rich countries are reachable within 36 hours from anywhere in the world, less time than the incubation period of many infectious diseases.[27] A Londoner infected with a novel pathogen today might be in Washington tomorrow, unknowingly transmitting the contagion to a person who, four hours later, passes it on to someone else in Toronto who, in turn, infects another traveller who lands in Beijing 20 hours later. Never before in human history have so many people been on the move over such great distances so quickly. Today, airlines carry ten times more passengers than they did four decades ago.[28]

***

A basic truth about pandemics is that they burn out if all the transmission paths from human to human are severed. If every person on the planet isolated, a pathogen would disappear (though if it was a zoonosis it could jump back to humans later). Obviously, universal isolation is unworkable, although more pragmatic degrees of isolation are possible, and have proved effective in preventing community spread of SARS-Cov-2. Ramification of contact lies at the opposite end of the spectrum. The more interconnected we are, the more we travel, the more time we spend in the company of others (if only fleetingly), the more the world becomes a global community—in other words, the greater the expansion of potential pathogenic transmission belts—the more likely it is that someone's exposure to a pathogen of animal origin in one part of the world this morning will become an embryonic pandemic by evening.

It is the characteristics of modernity, then, that represent the great pandemic risk factors. The greater the world's population, the more vectors for a pathogen of animal origin to jump the species barrier to humans. The more ways there are for humans to connect with each other at home and around the globe, the more potential transmission belts there are for pathogens to engulf humanity.

Another aspect of modernity that increases pandemic risk is research on viruses, bacteria, and other pathogens that have the potential to mushroom into pandemics—so called potential pandemic pathogens, or PPPs. There is a paradox here. The research is conducted to help prevent and combat future pandemics. But at the same time, it increases the risk of pandemics, as mammograms—a tool used to detect breast cancer—increase the risk of malignancies.

Scientists around the world collect live samples of animal pathogens and bring them back to the laboratory for study. Sometimes they manipulate the pathogens genetically with the aim of making them infectious to humans to understand what characteristics pathogens must have to vault the species barrier. The purpose is to learn as much as possible about potential pandemic pathogens to gain knowledge that will help prevent and combat future outbreaks and guide vaccine development.

There are more than 200 lab facilities in the United States alone expressly built to safely contain the dangerous microbes with which scientists work, including drug-resistant tuberculosis, influenza, coronaviruses, plague, anthrax, botulism, ricin, and Ebola, among others. In 2012, over forty of these facilities were engaged in researching live PPPs—that is, active microbial agents that if accidentally introduced into the community could spark an outbreak of global magnitude. And that's only in the United States. Similar facilities exist in many other countries around the world.

Research on pathogens always carries risks. Scientists can become infected accidentally by animals when collecting disease-causing microbes in the field or through mishaps in the laboratory. They may not know they're infected, and unwittingly transmit the pathogen to their co-workers, friends, or family, setting off a chain of infections that eventually engulfs the world. The risks cannot be blithely dismissed as trivial.

To be sure, the laboratories in which the most dangerous diseases are studied are custom built for containment, and stringent safety protocols are followed to prevent accidents from happening. All the same, accidents do happen. And though the likelihood of an accident happening in a single lab in a single year may be quite small, over many years and many labs, the chance of at least one accident occurring approaches certainty.

Assume, for the sake of illustration, that the probability of a live pathogen escaping from a single lab in 12 months is a meager three tenths of one percent. Lab workers can feel a justifiable sense of assurance about their safety—and that of the public. But with 42 labs in the United States carrying out research with live potential pandemic of pathogens, there is an 80 percent chance of a leak from one or more these labs every 13 years.[29] Add all the other labs in the world that carry out similar research, and the odds of a lab-leak happening at some point become even more likely.

Imagine playing Russian Roulette with one bullet in a gun with one hundred chambers. Chances are very good that if you play a few rounds, you'll survive. But if a thousand people play the same game many times, it's all but certain that for at least one of them, the game will end badly.

Considering that we're living with "a global proliferation of high-containment biological laboratories"—the equivalent of a growing number of people playing Russian Roulette—the chance of a lab-leak is virtually certain. Ever since 9/11 enkindled fears of bio-terrorism, countries have gone on a laboratory building spree.[30] It's no surprise, then, to find that lab leaks are not a theoretical phenomenon. They actually occur. And in frighteningly large numbers.

Over a seven year period ending in 2013, US labs averaged over 200 safety incidents per year. These mishaps were serious enough to be reported to federal authorities. On average, over 100 US lab workers are treated or monitored as a result of safety lapses every year. There have been accidents involving anthrax, Ebola, and bird flu at the Centers for Disease Control and Prevention, the mishandling of smallpox virus at the National Institutes of Health, and the accidental shipping of live virus from a US military lab to allied military bases around the world.

Six incidents involving lab-manipulated coronaviruses at the University of North Carolina were reported to US safety officials from January 1, 2015, through June 1, 2020.[31] Meanwhile, the United States Army Medical Research Institute of Infectious Diseases at Fort Detrick—established after World War II to continue the biowarfare research begun by German and Japanese scientists—has been shut down on numerous occasions for safety violations.

In 2004, a researcher at the National Institute of Virology in Beijing accidentally infected herself with the virus that causes SARS. She unwittingly transmitted the virus to others, including her mother, who died. In 2012, a scientist engaged in vaccine research at a California medical center died after he inadvertently infected himself with live Neisseria meningitides bacteria. There's even speculation that the H1N1 flu strain that resurfaced in 1977 was "probably an accidental release from a laboratory source," according to a 2009 article in the New England Journal of Medicine.[32] And these incidents are only the tip of the iceberg. With a pandemic-like growth in the number of labs doing research on dangerous pathogens worldwide, the chance that an accidental leak from a lab will trigger an outbreak is a near certainty.

This raises a question: Is the quest for knowledge about PPPs as foolhardy as looking for a gas leak with a lit match? Some scientists think it is. They say the consequences of an accidental spillover of a pathogen from the laboratory to an immunologically naïve human population could be profound—health systems overwhelmed, deep economic crisis, and possibly tens, if not hundreds, of millions of people dead. The probability of a potential pandemic-initiating lab leak is too large to ignore.

Lab accidents ought to be considered a major pandemic risk factor, along with population growth, growing population density, and increasing interconnectedness. Oddly, they're not. That is, unless the labs are located in China. Despite the large number of PPP labs in the United States, and notwithstanding their chequered safety record, only Chinese labs were considered in the US orbit among government officials and mainstream media as a possible source of the Covid-19 outbreak. This reflected a chauvinist political bias. Lab accidents can, and do, happen outside of China, including in the United States. If a lab leak was going to be considered as a possible source of the outbreak, mishaps in any lab conducting research with coronaviruses should have been considered, not just the Chinese labs.

Lab accidents as a pandemic risk factor were politicized—and on a number of levels. One level was geopolitical. In an effort to vilify China—part of an ongoing low-level war against the Communist-led country—the US government attempted to frame Covid-19 as a Chinese disease. Persuading the world that Chinese malfeasance was responsible for the novel coronavirus suited US foreign policy goals admirably. The targets of the US accusations were two Wuhan virology labs. The US government and various commentators pointed to the possibility that SARS-Cov-2 leaked from one of these labs. There was no evidence, but US president Joe Biden, following the previous Trump administration, ordered the US intelligence community to look for indications, recalling George W. Bush's sham inquiry into whether Iraq had weapons of mass destruction.

Yanzhong Huang, a senior fellow for global health at the Council on Foreign Relations, wrote an editorial in *The Washington Post* in June of 2021, titled "China could pay if nations come to believe the virus leaked from a lab." Huang's organization, the Council on Foreign Relations, is a Wall Street-funded and -directed think tank that provides policy advice to the State Department. It is firmly interlocked with the US foreign policy establishment and the Biden administration. Typically, members of the council fill top cabinet positions. Biden's secretaries of state, treasury, defense, and commerce were members, as were the UN ambassador, the national security advisor, CIA director, Indo-Pacific czar, and chief of staff, among others.

Huang's editorial noted that China had "enjoyed prestige on the world stage for its containment of the pandemic, especially compared with many Western countries" but added that "if missteps by Chinese scientists" were seen to be "the cause of that pandemic, such praise would quickly fade." "Even a belief in a coverup without firm evidence of wrongdoing would be damaging," he wrote. Moreover, if US intelligence was seen as exposing a coverup, it could re-establish the United States' "reputation for competence," badly tarnished by the country's dismal performance in managing the Covid-19 pandemic.

Huang counseled that fostering a belief in a Chinese coverup— even if there was no evidence of one— would:

- "Precipitate a free fall in China's relationship with the outside world";
- Provide a pretext for the United States to boycott the 2022 Beijing Winter Olympics;
- Raise questions in China about whether the Communist Party is fit to rule;
- Force China to close in on itself in a fit of angry isolation as it is shunned by the rest of the world.

In other words, there were strong *raisons d'État* for Washington— which made no secret of reviling China as an enemy to be contained and countered—to manufacture a belief in a coverup.

A number of scientists, some of whom had legitimate concerns about the risks of PPP research, played into Washington's anti-China designs, signing an open letter calling on the WHO to revisit its investigation into the origins of the novel coronavirus. The

WHO investigation had concluded that the virus likely originated in bats and spread to an unidentified second species before spilling over into humans, and that a spillover through a laboratory accident was highly unlikely. The scientists called for a new inquiry to consider five possible pathways, all but one of which, if found to be the cause, would implicate Wuhan lab scientists or technicians.

The authors listed the following as the possible origins of the virus.

- A pure zoonosis event;
- Infection at a sampling site of a lab employee or accompanying non-lab personnel;
- Infection during transport of collected animals or samples;
- Infection acquired in a lab;
- Viral escape from a lab.

The politicized nature of the call for a reinvestigation was revealed in the fact that the investigation's scope of inquiry was restricted to the two Wuhan labs. The investigation would not ask:

- Did the novel coronavirus originate in an incident at another lab, including any based in the United States?
- Are the risks of research on potential pandemic pathogens acceptable?

Under pressure from Washington, the WHO proposed a second investigation. Among other steps, the WHO announced it would conduct "audits of relevant laboratories and research institutions operating in the area of the initial human cases identified in December 2019"—namely, Wuhan. Audits were not planned for laboratories outside China that were also conducting research on coronaviruses and could possibly have experienced a safety failure. The WHO said it expected "China to support this next phase of the scientific process by sharing all relevant data in a spirit of transparency," while at the same time bidding "all Member States" to refrain

"from politicising" the investigation. That hope was naïve if not dis-
ingenuous. The WHO itself politicized the proposed inquiry when
it declared that "finding where this virus came from [is] important
as an obligation to the families of the [then] 4 million people who
[had] lost someone they love, and the millions who have suffered."[33]
If an inquiry found that SARS-CoV-2 leaked from a Wuhan laboratory, China would be held responsible for four million deaths. This
would shift blame for hundreds of thousands of US deaths from
Washington's outstandingly poor pandemic performance to China.

Beijing had understandable concerns about the second investigation. It was clear that Washington had no sincere interest in
the origins of the pandemic—or in the larger question of whether
the risks of research with potential pandemic pathogens are too
great—and was only interested in promoting discourse about China
as the pandemic's culprit.

With the lab leak question now thoroughly politicized, it was
impossible to broach the matter of whether the proliferation of
biological laboratories worldwide was putting humanity at greater
risk of future pandemics. Any discussion of the matter was vehemently opposed by Beijing and its supporters on the grounds that it
was a cover for legitimizing the innuendo Washington was making
about the novel coronavirus spilling out of a Wuhan lab. On the
other hand, promoters of the Wuhan lab innuendo glommed on
to any discussion of the risks of collecting pathogens in the wild
and bringing them back to the lab, but narrowly focused it on the
Wuhan laboratories, dismissing peremptorily any discussion of
the dangers of comparable research in labs outside of China or
the question of whether the pandemic could have originated in an
accident in one of several US labs engaged in coronavirus research.

In the United States there were also countervailing institutional
biases that discouraged questions about whether lab work with
potential zoonotic pathogens constituted a major risk factor for
future pandemics.

There is a community of specialists in infectious diseases,
comprising immunologists, vaccine experts, pharmacologists, and

epidemiologists. This community concerns itself with the collection and study of potential pandemic pathogens, as well as treatments and vaccines against them. It is also this community that is looked to, to identify pandemic risk factors. Many of the people in this community either depend for their employment on research with hazardous microbes at any of the expanding number of biological labs throughout the world, or oversee such research.

Anthony Fauci, the veteran head of the National Institute of Allergy and Infectious Diseases in the United States, "oversees an extensive portfolio of basic and applied research to prevent, diagnose, and treat established infectious diseases," according to the NIAID website. The research Fauci superintends is carried out at numerous labs, including the Wuhan Institute of Virology. Fauci was elevated in the public mind as the leading figure in the Western world on the novel coronavirus pandemic. If "the science" that was often invoked by politicians to justify their pandemic-related decisions was personified, that person would be Fauci. "Dr. Science" would be a fitting moniker for the feisty physician turned bureaucrat. The moniker is no less fitting considering that Fauci, himself, sees himself as science personified. "I represent science," he declared, adding that anyone who criticized him was "really criticizing science."[34] It's unlikely that Dr. Science could identify lab mishaps as major pandemic risk factors. As the novelist Upton Sinclair once quipped, "It's difficult to get a man to understand something when his salary depends on his not understanding it."[35] The same might be said of the countless infectious disease researchers who make their living collecting pathogens in the wild and studying them in the lab, funded by Fauci's NIAID.

A Stanford microbiologist told journalist and author Nina Burleigh that, like anyone else, scientists are reluctant to own up to their mistakes.

> If there had been a laboratory accident, think about what the consequences might be. If there were evidence that a benign accident, let's say [by the] Wuhan Institute of Virology, led to this world pandemic and millions of deaths, every one of my colleagues and

peers [in] science knows this could have huge, grave consequences for how we view the conduct of science in laboratories working on infectious agents. It has huge consequence for how we fund science, for oversight, for how decisions are made about what we're going to do and not do.[36]

Scientists involved in infectious disease research are, for reasons related less to science and more to their livelihoods, inclined to favor explanations of the origin of SARS-Cov-2 that deny the possibility of lab-related accidents. Questioning what goes on in laboratories staffed by phalanxes of Ph.Ds seems ... well, anti-science.

But what many people construe as science, is not science at all, but its trappings: test tubes, beakers, lab coats, microscopes, vials, syringes. Charlatans peddle their nostrums by exploiting the association of science with the objects to which science has become inextricably linked. Grifters without medical degrees don lab coats, wrap stethoscopes around their necks, and utter multisyllabic Latin words, to beguile credulous customers into buying quack cures. Chiropractors, posing as science-based practitioners, manipulate spines to cure disease by correcting "vital forces"—pure flummery, based on not a jot of science. Many people erroneously believe that chiropractors are back doctors—specialists in the treatment of lower back pain. Although they surround themselves with an aura of scientific legitimacy, chiropractors are, in point of fact, quacks who are quite happy to pose as the back specialists they are not. Physiotherapists trot out an array of seemingly impressive technology, including therapeutic ultrasound, for which there's not one iota of evidence that any of it works. A random control study conducted by Britain's National Health Service found that patients who underwent a course of physiotherapy for back pain took longer to recover than patients who were given a set of exercises to do at home.[37] The science in this is not the ultrasound wands that physiotherapists wave over aching backs to no effect, but the NHS random control study to find out whether physiotherapy and its seemingly impressive technology make any difference.

Science is not technology; it is a method of inquiry based on careful observation and application of logic to evidence. Vaccines are no more a scientific way of combatting a pandemic than are stay-at-home orders and mask-wearing. True, vaccines are a *product* of the scientific method, but so too are toasters. We wouldn't say a breakfast consisting of two slices of toast is scientific, because a toaster is involved. Science is simply a way of answering questions. For example, the question of whether a strategy of mass vaccination is more or less effective than non-pharmaceutical public health measures in stopping community spread of a highly infectious disease can be answered scientifically. If we observe that countries that rely on old-school epidemiological measures are more successful in shielding their citizens from a pathogen than countries that rely mainly on mass vaccination, we've engaged in science if we conclude that public health measures are likely more effective. The conclusion is based on inference from careful observation. That's science. In contrast, if we declare a mass vaccination campaign to be the best approach to combatting Covid-19 because vaccines are based on science, we are making an unscientific and meaningless statement, on par with pronouncing penicillin the best treatment for a broken limb because penicillin is based on science.

Neither is technology inherently good owing to its scientific connection. Consider nuclear reactors. They are the outcome of centuries of careful observation and application of logic by countless scientists. Most people would acknowledge that discussing whether the risks of nuclear power are tolerable given the devastating consequences of accidents is not anti-scientific. However, the question of whether the risks of laboratory research with potential pandemic pathogens are tolerable in light of the devastating consequences of accidents has been stigmatized as against science. Indeed, the question has become taboo in some circles, discouraging any effort to identify PPP research as a risk factor for future pandemics.

Two factors, then, militated against recognition of PPP research as a pandemic risk factor. The first was Washington's attempt to blame China for the Covid-19 pandemic, by insinuating the idea into public discourse that SARS-Cov-2 leaked from a Wuhan lab. China and its supporters flatly rejected any discussion of the dangers of PPP research on the grounds that the discussion was a cover for focusing public attention of the Wuhan Virology Institute as the source of a possible lab accident. Beijing's concerns were not without foundation. Washington and its supporters were happy to discuss the dangers of PPP research, but only as they related to the Wuhan lab, brooking no discussion of the dangers of PPP research generally or acknowledging that if it was possible that an accident at a Wuhan lab triggered the novel coronavirus pandemic, then so too was it possible that an accident at a US (or some other country's) lab did the same.

The second set of factors was a taboo against questioning any enterprise that surrounded itself with an aura of scientific legitimacy, along with the institutional bias of the infectious disease community against acknowledging, for fear of losing jobs and funding, that PPP research may bear risks too large to tolerate. The question of whether the risks are intolerably large ought to be one for the public to decide, not scientists. We wouldn't entrust the assessment of how tolerable the risks of nuclear power are to nuclear engineers and nuclear physicists; nor should we entrust assessments about the acceptability of PPP research risks to PPP researchers.

***

While it's often said that pandemics are inevitable, it's more accurate to say they're highly likely, and their high degree of likelihood is inherent in the nature of modernity. Snowden observed that "COVID-19 flared up and spread because it is suited to the society we have made. A world with nearly eight billion people, the majority of whom live in densely crowded cities all linked by rapid air travel, creates innumerable opportunities for pulmonary viruses."[38] Population growth, increasing population density, growing interconnectedness, and the dangers of pathogens escaping accidentally from labs—all these factors predispose humanity to future pandemics. But if new pathogens are highly likely to emerge in the future, is it also true that pandemics are inevitable? In other words, does the emergence of a novel pathogen automatically equal tragedy?

CHAPTER 2

THE RESPONSE

"To me, this feels honestly more about economics than about the science." — Yonatan Grad, Associate Professor of Immunology and Infectious Diseases, Harvard University[1]

"COVID-19 remains a global disaster. Worse it was a preventable disaster." — WHO Independent Expert Panel[2]

Pandemics are not inevitable.

To be sure, the emergence of new infectious diseases is a near certainty. Pathogenesis—the birth of a new disease—is a necessary condition of pandemics, but it is not a sufficient condition. That pandemics are optional and not inevitable is provable by reference to one word: China. By following a zero-Covid strategy of eliminating local transmission of the novel coronavirus, the Communist-led country avoided overwhelmed hospitals, limited fatalities to extraordinarily low levels, and escaped significant economic hardship. While the pandemic danced a macabre waltz around it, China, along with a handful of other countries that followed a similar strategy, failed to show up at the ball.

Public discourse outside China and other zero-Covid countries accepted the pandemic as an inevitability. The narrative was highly influenced by people such as billionaire Bill Gates, who advanced the view that pandemics are unavoidable, and that vaccines and drug therapies should be developed in anticipation of their ineluctable arrival. CEPI, the Center for Epidemic Preparedness and Innovation—a non-profit organization that played a leading role in the fight against Covid-19 among countries in the US orbit—was born as a vehicle for promoting Gates' views and approach to emerging infectious diseases. Needless to say, the reality that the emergence of a novel pathogen is not a sufficient condition for a pandemic, and the fact that China demonstrated that a pandemic could be avoided by using mass testing, contact tracing, and isolation to break the chain of pathogenic transmission, refutes Gates' view.

While Gates is a major funder of the World Health Organization, the organization's director-general, Tedros Adhanom Ghebreyesus, rejected the erroneous Gates idea that vaccines ought to be the principal tool used to fight pandemics. "Vaccines are not the only tool," Tedros announced. "Indeed, there is no single tool that will defeat the pandemic. We can only defeat it with a comprehensive approach of vaccines in combination with *proven* public health and social measures that *we know work*." (emphasis added).[3]

On the same day Tedros told the world it would need to combine vaccines with non-pharmaceutical public health measures to beat Covid-19, Eric Lander, US president Joe Biden's science adviser, promulgated a different view. He wrote in *The Washington Post* that "Coronavirus vaccines can end the current pandemic." Lander made his prediction at a time vaccines were available to any US adult who wanted one, but when US case counts—already high by world standards—were climbing. The vaccine strategy clearly *wasn't* working, though Lander appeared not to notice. Ignoring the reality that the United States' own experience impugned the ability of vaccines alone to end the pandemic, Lander—a multimillionaire who had substantial investments in the pharmaceutical industry—announced that "the scientific community has been developing a bold plan to keep future viruses from becoming pandemics." Would it involve the proven public health and social measures Tedros said we know work and that China had demonstrated do work?

No. Instead, it would be based on vaccines—the tool wealthy US Americans with stakes in drug companies, like Gates and Lander, continued to tout as the pathway of escape from pandemics, current and future. In the United States, and the countries that orbit the imperial center, all belief was for vaccines as the main route out of the pandemic, and all evidence was against.

The US government, according to Lander's plan, would see to it that vaccines were designed, tested, and approved within 100 days of detecting a new pandemic threat and would arrange to manufacture enough doses to supply the world within 200 days.[4] The folly of the approach was evident. First, there is no guarantee that effective vaccines can be developed for every pathogen, let alone in 100 days. There is no vaccine for AIDS, for example, despite the decades of effort scientists have invested in trying to develop one. Second, it's impossible to test a vaccine for safety in 100 days. Since the very short testing window allows scientists to follow test subjects only over a very brief period, it would be impossible to say whether the vaccine was free from any but immediate adverse side-effects. This would pose an enormous health risk to the billions of people who would be inoculated, perhaps greater than the risk of the novel pathogen itself. Third, even if the extraordinarily ambitious goal of manufacturing enough doses to supply the world within 200 days was met, the logistical difficulties of administering the vaccine to billions of people worldwide would take more than 200 days to overcome; it would likely take years.

In the meantime, the only way to prevent the pandemic pathogen from running out of control, killing millions, collapsing healthcare systems, and devastating economies, would be to implement the proven public health and social measures we know work. It would seem, then, that the best way of meeting the challenge of future pandemics is, in the first instance, to figure out why most countries failed to implement the proven public health and social measures that could have prevented the Covid-19 pandemic, so that the impediments that blocked an effective response can be overcome the next time the world confronts a novel pathogen. Why was a strategy that worked in China, South Korea, and New Zealand, as well as in Vietnam and North Korea, rejected everywhere else?

Despite China having every pandemic risk factor, it was one of the few countries that escaped a Covid-19 catastrophe. It has the world's largest population, close to one hundred cities with populations of one million or more, high-speed trains to whisk passengers from one part of the country to another, innumerable airline connections to the rest of the world, and yes, scientists who collect coronaviruses from the wild and study them in laboratories. All the same, China was not struck by disaster. The numbers of infections and deaths per million were held to astonishingly low levels, the healthcare system did not collapse, and economic activity recovered quickly. What's more, China may very well have been ground zero for the virus. It was the first country to identify the new infection—and while that doesn't mean the virus originated there—there's a good chance it did. And yet the Communist-led country emerged almost unscathed. If ever there were an answer to the question of whether pathogenic catastrophes are optional, China is it.

**

In May 2021, more than a year into the pandemic, the World Health Organization released a report by an independent panel on the performance of the world's governments in responding to the Covid-19 health emergency.[5] The panel arrived at a stunning conclusion. The pandemic could have been avoided. It wasn't inevitable, even as late as January 30, 2020, the day the WHO declared a public health emergency of international concern, and two to three months after the virus likely first began to circulate. Even at this late date it was "still possible to interrupt virus spread, provided that countries put in place strong measures to detect disease early, isolate and treat cases, trace contacts and promote social distancing measures commensurate with the risk." But that didn't happen. By March 11, 2020, the virus had spread far enough that the global health organization declared a pandemic. How had an avoidable pandemic become a catastrophe on a world scale?

The answer was simple. Inaction. "On 30 January 2020, it should have been clear to all countries from the declaration of the" public health emergency of international concern "that COVID-19 represented a serious threat," the panel stated. "Even so," it continued, "only a minority of countries set in motion comprehensive and coordinated Covid-19 protection and response measures." The result was that February 2020, a month "when steps could and should have been taken to" prevent a controllable outbreak from irrupting into a pandemic, was lost to history. Governments tarried, and their foot-dragging plunged the world into the dark abyss of a pulmonary pandemic.

Not all governments were content to sit tight until it was absolutely certain they were staring disaster in the face. "China, New Zealand, Republic of Korea, Singapore and Thailand and Viet Nam," the panel noted, all acted quickly and decisively to contain the emergency, and all with exemplary success. These countries, the panel reported, pursued an aggressive containment strategy that involved mass testing, robust contact tracing, and quarantine, with "social and economic support to promote widespread uptake of public health measures."

While the panel failed to mention North Korea, the East Asian country also acted swiftly, sealing its borders on January 21, even before the WHO declared a global health emergency. The country's leader, Kim Jong Un, called pandemic control North Korea's "top priority" and "most important work."[6] The Washington Post noted that Pyongyang had taken the pandemic "hyper-seriously,"[7] while The New York Times observed that "North Korea has taken some of the most drastic actions of any country against the virus."[8] These reports accorded with the country's claim to have experienced not a single Covid-19 case. Howard Waitzkin, a physician with a Ph.D. in sociology, critically examined North Korea's Covid-19 claims, concluding that Pyongyang's report of zero cases and zero deaths "is plausible" and the DPRK may, in fact, have led the world in the fight against COVID-19.[9]

Most other countries, by contrast, waited far too long to act. And when they did act, they failed to do enough, never fully implementing the measures needed to bring their outbreaks under control. What's more, they almost invariably dialed back measures too soon, with catastrophic consequences for the health of their citizens.

"Countries with the poorest results," the panel found, "had uncoordinated approaches that devalued science, denied the potential impact of the pandemic, delayed comprehensive action, and allowed distrust to undermine efforts. Many had health systems beset by long-standing problems of fragmentation, undervaluing of health workers and underfunding."

So, why did most countries do too little, too late? The panel pointed to cost. Most governments judged concerted public health action—the aggressive test, trace, and isolate measures implemented by China and a handful of other countries—as too expensive. Three costs were central to their concerns:

- The direct expense of testing, contact tracing, the construction of isolation facilities, coordinating quarantine, and providing financial support to the quarantined.
- The indirect cost of business disruptions.
- The impact on the stock market.

Concerning the first cost, according to best-selling author Michael Lewis's study of the US response to the Covid-19 pandemic, *The Premonition: A Pandemic Story,* the "people inside the American government who would be charged with executing various aspects of any pandemic strategy ... believed none of these so-called non-pharmaceutical interventions"—the kind China pursued to great effect—"would contribute anything but economic loss."[10]

Concerning the cost of business disruption, the Great Influenza offered an anticipatory model. Studies of how the United States responded to the 1918-1920 flu pandemic found that government decision-makers were under incessant pressure from businesses to lift public health measures. Now as then, capitalist governments were highly influenced by business communities and finely attuned to their needs. Minimizing the cost to business was the top priority of governments working out how to deal with a global health crisis.

Finally, US president Donald Trump deliberately downplayed the public health emergency, repeatedly declaring that it would magically resolve itself, because he feared that acknowledging the danger would result in untold stock market losses.[11] "Trump grew concerned that any [strong] action by his administration would hurt the economy, and ... told advisers that he [did] not want the administration to do or say anything that would ... spook the markets," reported *The Washington Post*.[12] What the WHO panel perceived as "a wait and see" attitude on the part of many governments was actually a "take no strong action to avoid spooking the markets" attitude. The contrast between China's aggressive response and the United States' "see, hear, and speak no evil" approach, is revealingly summarized in the comments of the countries' respective leaders: China's Xi Jinping: "Infectious disease control is not merely a matter of public health and hygiene; it's an all-encompassing issue and a total war"; the United States' Donald Trump: "One day—it's like a miracle—it will disappear."[13]

***

China's success in protecting the health of its citizens from the ravages of Covid-19 was perhaps the greatest public health accomplishment in human history. By contrast, the United States' dismal Covid-19 performance was perhaps one of the greatest public health failures of all time.

Despite the fact that the first Covid-19 cases were identified in China, and the country's population is over four times the size of that of the United States, the number of confirmed Covid-19 cases in the United States surpassed China as early as March 26, 2020, only two weeks after the World Health Organization declared a pandemic. By March 29, US deaths due to Covid-19 had already inched past China's, and would continue to climb, with the gap between the two countries unremittingly increasing. The disparity between the US and Chinese figures—little mentioned in Western public discourse—was astonishing. By December 31, 2021, some 23 months after Chinese authorities reported a cluster of unusual pneumonia cases in Wuhan, there were nearly 55 million confirmed cases of Covid-19 in the United States, compared to slightly over 100,000 in the far more populous China. The number of people that had tested positive for Covid-19 was over 164,000 per million in the United States compared to only 71 per million in China. Incredibly, deaths per million in the United States were over 770 times greater than in China. Over 800,000 US Americans had died from Covid-19, making the outbreak the greatest death event, measured in absolute numbers of deaths, in US history, exceeding fatalities from World War I, World War II, the Korean War, the Vietnam War, the Great Influenza of 1918-1920, and even the Civil War. Meanwhile, in China, fewer than 5,000 had died, less than six-tenths of one percent of the US figure. At 3.2 people per million, Covid-19 deaths in China were less than two-tenths of one percent of the United States' 2,480 deaths per million. When it came to pandemic control, China and the United States inhabited different planets.

Was China the anomaly or was the United States? In fact, both were, though compared to the world at large, China performed anomalously better and the United States anomalously worse. On December 31, 2021, confirmed cases per million were over 500 times better in China than the world average and over four times worse than the world average in the United States. Confirmed deaths per million were over 200 times better in China but over three and a half times worse in the United States. The United States, with only four percent of the world's population, accounted for 19 percent of cases and 15 percent of deaths, while China, comprising 18 percent of the world's population, accounted for less than one-tenth of one percent of the world's cases and a similarly infinitesimal fraction of the world's deaths.[14]

The United States' utter failure by comparison with China, and failure even by comparison with the world at large, was a taboo subject, judging by the virtual absence of discussion of the numbers, despite the fact that the figures were readily available for inspection by anyone with access to the Internet. Our World in Data, a collaborative effort between researchers at the University of Oxford and the non-profit organization Global Change Data Lab, assembled a vast storehouse of Covid-19 information by country, from morbidity and mortality figures, to vaccine uptake statistics, and more. The yawning chasm between Washington and Beijing in pandemic performance was immediately evident to anyone who cared to inspect the data. No country or jurisdiction, with the exception of a handful of sparsely populated nations, had accumulated fewer cases or deaths per million than China. By comparison, the United States' record was among the worst in the world. All the same, journalists and academics in the US orbit mainly avoided Sino-US comparisons, and, on the rare occasions they did make comparisons, grossly understated the disparity. By avoiding quantitative comparisons, or obscuring them when they were made, the Western media prevented important questions from being asked. Why had China performed so much better, not only in comparison to the United States, but relative to virtually every other country in the world? Why hadn't China's approach, a manifest success, been emulated except by a few other countries? How many lives might have been saved had governments learned from the experience of the East Asian colossus?

Washington failed in multiple ways.

- To avoid spooking the markets and to preserve investor wealth, it refused to acknowledge the seriousness of the threat.
- It refused to emulate the successful approach of China to stop the outbreak, rejecting non-pharmaceutical pandemic control measures as too costly.
- It eschewed successful non-pharmaceutical pandemic control measures, even after it became unavoidably clear that China's

approach was the most effective way to safeguard the health of US citizens.

These failures precipitated a pandemic and produced avoidable death on a scale never before seen in US history. How many lives were needlessly sacrificed to the stock market and Washington's desire to spare the business community the expense and inconveniences of public health measures?

It's possible to answer this question. Had Washington emulated China's approach, an estimated 1,067 US Americans would have died from Covid-19 by December 31, 2021 (equivalent to the number of Covid-19 deaths per million China experienced, adjusted to the size of the US population). That is 823,173 fewer deaths than the actual US Covid-19 death toll to that date. In other words, to protect the stock market and avoid the costs of implementing stringent non-pharmaceutical public health measures, the lives of more than 800,000 US Americans were sacrificed. Had Canada emulated the Chinese approach, an estimated 122 Canadians would have died from Covid-19, compared to over 30,000 that actually did die. In the United Kingdom, 216 would have died compared to more than 146,000 whose lives were cut short by London's failed pandemic response.

What if the world as a whole had followed China's lead? Had that happened, an estimated 25,239 people would have died from Covid-19 by December 31, 2021, compared to over 5,428,000 that actually did perish, a difference of over 5,402,000 people. The failure of the world's governments to act in a manner that China, early on, had demonstrated was an effective means of controlling the outbreak, created in excess of 5.4 million preventable deaths, some two years after the world became aware of the novel coronavirus.

***

Infectious disease management strategies are guided by one or more of the following goals:

- To minimize the health burden on the community—that is, to achieve the lowest possible level of sickness and mortality. As we've seen from China's experience, it was possible to keep morbidity and mortality to very low levels, using methods Tedros called "proven" and "known to work."
- To limit sickness so that it does not impose an undue burden on hospitals and other healthcare resources.
- To minimize disruptions to the economy and the accumulation of profit.

These goals are complementary in some ways and contradictory in others. The goal of minimizing illness and mortality is consistent with the goal of minimizing the burden on hospitals. On the other hand, hospital capacity may be large enough to accommodate morbidity and mortality at levels above an achievable minimum. The goal of managing infection levels to the maximum tolerable limit of hospital capacity therefore may contradict the goal of minimizing the health burden on the community. While it is possible to drive infection levels to near zero, and while it is known that this possibility exists, most governments tolerated infection levels higher than this, allowing infection levels to rise to limits tolerable within healthcare budgets. The goal, then, was not to minimize deaths, but to minimize disruptions to the economy by allowing infections to rise to the maximum level hospitals could tolerate.

Calibrating infection levels to hospital capacity and healthcare resources may appear to mesh closely with the goal of minimizing disruptions to the economy. The key word is "appear." It is very likely that decision-makers in most governments assumed, in the days prior to vaccines becoming available, that the goal of minimizing the health burden on the community was antithetical to minimizing disruptions to the economy, although, as we'll see, the assumption was wrong. It's also likely that most governments were under pressure to meet the third goal (minimizing disruptions to the economy and profit accumulation), but were compelled, for the sake of avoiding an escalating health emergency, to try to limit the burden enough—but only enough—that the hospitals and health-care systems they managed did not collapse.

Outside of China, public health officials, epidemiologists, and infectious disease specialists assumed that the world would eventually arrive at a state where the virus burned itself out and the burden on healthcare systems would become manageable. At that point, the public health emergency, or pandemic, would be over, and Covid-19 would become endemic—that is, SARS-CoV-2 would continue to circulate, but would, on any given day, hospitalize so few people that the burden on healthcare systems would be readily accommodated within current budgets. The key question was how to arrive at this point without, in the interim, overwhelming hospitals and overstretching medical resources.

The view throughout much of the world, influenced strongly by the United States, was that a vaccine would be the exit ramp from the pandemic. Eventually, it was hoped, safe and effective vaccines would prevent enough people from becoming seriously ill that the burden on healthcare resources would be readily managed. But what if developing a safe and effective vaccine quickly was beyond current competencies? Not all attempts to produce vaccines are successful. For example, despite decades of trying, a vaccine has never been developed for AIDS. What's more, even if efforts to produce a vaccine proved successful, how long would it take? Until inoculations against Covid-19 came along, vaccines normally took many years to develop—a half decade or longer. A vaccine might be the cavalry that never arrived, or arrived long after the virus had spread so widely that most people had either died or acquired immunity through infection. These realities raise questions about why so much faith was placed in a vaccine savior when, from the juncture the World Health Organization declared a public health emergency of global concern early in 2020, any reasonable person would have concluded that vaccines were a huge gamble. Indeed, any reasonable person would have also wondered why the dice were being rolled on a vaccine, when a proven and effective way to eliminate community transmission of the virus—demonstrated by China and a few other countries—was already at hand. That vaccines were actually developed in record time, is beside the point. At the time, no one knew whether the seemingly Herculean task of developing effective vaccines in 12 months was achievable. Moreover, even if it were possible to know in advance that the vaccine gamble would pay off, the question of how healthcare systems would be protected in the interim, would still need to be answered.

Governments followed one or more of the following strategies to achieve one or more of the three goals noted above.

- Elimination, also known as no community transmission, zero-Covid, or crushing the curve.
- Mitigation, sometimes called hospital surveillance-based mitigation, controlled transmission, bending the curve, or flattening the curve.
- No mitigation, known also as uncontrolled transmission, or living with Covid.

The first two strategies were pursued by non-pharmaceutical interventions, or NPIs. NPIs seek to disrupt the chain of viral transmission from infected to uninfected individuals, mainly by reducing person to person contact. NPIs include stay-at-home and work-at-home orders, prohibitions on mass gatherings, the closure of schools and non-essential businesses, physical distancing, improved ventilation, and the wearing of masks. NPIs also involve isolation. Whole communities can be closed off from the rest of the world through rigorous border controls, to prevent the importation of infections from other countries. Additionally, infected individuals can be isolated within the community to prevent their transmitting the virus to other people. Isolating infected individuals means first identifying them, by means of testing, and then tracing their contacts, and testing their contacts, as well. Once identified, infected individuals and their contacts can be quarantined until they are no longer a danger to the community.

Pharmaceutical interventions include vaccines and drug therapies. While optimism prevailed early on that drugs could be developed to treat Covid-19 patients, successes were largely limited to vaccines. That's not to say that therapies weren't developed or found. They were. The steroid dexamethasone proved effective in treating hospitalized patients with severe cases. The antiviral drug, Remdesivir, was used to treat hospitalized patients. Monoclonal antibody therapies, developed by Regeneron and GlaxoSmithKline, were available for use with patients who weren't ill enough to be hospitalized. Merck and Pfizer developed antiviral pills for patients with mild to moderate disease.

Vaccines have their greatest role in mitigation and uncontrolled transmission scenarios. While they have a place in elimination strategies, they are redundant under a zero-Covid scenario, since elimination drives infection rates to zero, or near zero. Vaccines do, however, have a role to play in elimination in allowing strict border controls—one of the principal features of the elimination strategy—to be gradually eased. Once most of the population is vaccinated and protected from serious illness, the dangers of imported infections are greatly reduced.

While SARS-CoV-2 can be virtually eliminated through vigorous zero-Covid measures, it cannot be eradicated, as small pox was in the twentieth century. Small pox had four characteristics that made its eradication possible. It wasn't present in other species, and therefore couldn't jump back to humans if the disease was expunged in the human population. It was readily identifiable. Small pox cases were unlikely to be mistaken for other diseases and therefore overlooked. As a result, small pox carriers could be isolated quickly. The disease, once called the "speckled monster," had a short period of infectiousness, and so was less contagious than many other transmissible diseases. Finally, immunity acquired by vaccine or infection lasted a lifetime.

By contrast, SARS-CoV-2 is present in other species. Even if the virus was eradicated in humans, it could jump back from bats, cats, rabbits, dogs, minks, white-tailed deer, and possibly other species, all of which host the virus. To eliminate the virus completely, it would be necessary to eliminate it in all other host species as well—an impossible task.

Another complication: Covid-19 has features that overlap other respiratory diseases. It can look like flu, pneumonia, or a bad cold. This is a reason why it's unclear whether Covid-19 first emerged in China. It could have originated elsewhere, but was misdiagnosed as any of a number of other respiratory diseases. Rather than being the site of the first Covid-19 case, China may have only been the site of the first Covid-19 *diagnosis*—not the same. Because Covid-19 resembles other respiratory disorders, it is more likely than small pox to be misidentified, and therefore more likely to evade control measures. Additionally, Covid-19 has a longer period of pre-symptomatic infectiousness than small pox, making it more likely that people infected with the disease will interact with friends, family, and co-workers, transmitting the virus to them, before the emergence of symptoms leads to isolation. What's more, some Covid-19 cases are asymptomatic—a condition inconducive to control measures. Finally, it's unclear whether immunity acquired by vaccine or infection lasts a lifetime. What is clear, however, is that the current set of Covid-19 vaccines do not prevent transmission. That means the virus can continue to circulate, even among people who have been vaccinated. For all these reasons, SARS-CoV-2 appears to be ineradicable.

***

The most common Covid-19 control strategy pursued by rich countries, including in parts of the United States, in Canada, and in the United Kingdom, was mitigation. Mitigation is a strategy of bending or flattening the curve. Unfortunately, the term "flatten the curve," while based on commonly used words, does more to conceal than clarify what the strategy actually seeks to accomplish.

The curve the mitigation strategy sets out to flatten is a line that describes the number of infections that would occur in a community over time if no measures were taken to limit the spread of the virus. Imagine that an infected person transmits the virus to two other people. (This is not quite what happens with Covid-19, but for the sake of illustration, let's assume it is.) On day one, one person has the disease. The next day, two more have it. The day after, four more people are infected. The number of new infections continues to double every day: 8, 16, 32, 64, 128, and so on. Growth accelerates. Soon hospitals are full. Resources available to handle the ill deplete as doctors, nurses, medical technicians, and paramedics become sick. Hospitals run out of oxygen to treat patients. Undeterred, the virus continues to spread.

But the virus can only spread to uninfected people. Locating immunologically naïve targets is easy at first. Almost everyone has no defense against the virus. But as the virus afflicts more people, the pool of potential victims drains. Eventually, the spread of the virus reaches an inflection point. The possibilities for new infections recede. Like a wild fire that has consumed most of the combustible material within its reach, the virus starts to burn out. The number of new infections falls by half each day, from 128 to 64 to 32 to 16 to 8 and so on.

This scenario can be graphed as a bell curve. The apex of the bell, or curve, represents the point at which the virus produces its greatest number of infections. If no measures are taken to control viral diffusion, this point will be reached fairly quickly, and it will be high. But once the apex is reached, case-loads fall quickly, and the crisis soon ends. Like removing a bandage rapidly, the pain is great, but brief.

Of course, this would never happen in real life. It is never the case that outbreaks are passively accepted. People react to the rapid spread of illness by taking steps to protect themselves. If they see a growing number of people around them falling ill, they limit their contacts, avoid crowds, isolate at home, wash their hands frequently, and don masks. Governments, too, react to pressure on hospitals and other healthcare resources. They invoke emergency public health measures to protect healthcare systems from collapse. Some form of mitigation is always present.

Bending the curve is a way of redrawing the theoretical bell curve by pushing on the top to flatten it out. Flattening the curve has a desirable consequence—the apex, the point at which infections per day reach their maximum, is reduced to a level manageable within current healthcare resources. But there's a cost. Slowing the spread of the virus to prevent its putting too much stress on medical systems means slowing the rate at which the virus attacks the vulnerable population. If the crisis ends only when most people acquire immunity through illness, then, absent a vaccine, the more the curve is bent, the longer it will take the virus to burn itself out. Hence, implicit in the mitigation strategy is the expectation that, for a highly infectious disease like Covid-19, most people will become ill eventually but that the spread of infection throughout the community will happen slowly. Under this strategy, infections aren't avoided; they're drawn out over a long enough period that the apex of the curve never exceeds the capacity of hospitals and other medical resources to care for the ill.

This may shock those who diligently followed public health orders, avoided large crowds, washed their hands frequently, and wore masks, thinking the purpose was to keep them safe while the virus was made to go away and the pandemic brought to an end. In fact, the purpose was to keep hospitals safe from a sudden cataract of Covid-19 patients. Eventually, most people get sick under a mitigation scenario—that is, until, or *if*, a vaccine comes along. Unless the transmissibility of a pathogen is low, and so will yield readily to containment measures, most people must become ill to build the immunity that is the indispensable condition of a health emergency reaching its terminal point. This reality is unavoidable. A pandemic only ends when most people acquire immunity through infection or vaccination. The goal of mitigation is to bring the pandemic to a close by calibrating the rate at which a population acquires immunity by infection to the capacity of medical resources to care for those who become ill enough to require hospitalization.

The way governments implemented mitigation in practice was to impose public health restrictions to reduce hospital admissions, and then to ease them when hospitalizations were significantly reduced. The lifting of restrictive measures inevitably led to a resurgence, whereupon public health measures were re-imposed. This cyclical process was dubbed hospital surveillance-based mitigation, since the decision to impose or withdraw public health restrictions depended on surveillance of the number of people admitted to hospital with Covid-19. The practice of alternately imposing and lifting mitigation measures produced a series of waves. The waves were the inevitable product of the mitigation strategy. But in public discourse, the waves were treated as natural phenomena beyond human control, like the tides. They were, on the contrary, the necessary outcome of calibrating sickness to the capacity of medical systems to accommodate it.

Once vaccines were developed and made widely available, some governments adopted a new strategy: living with Covid. The new strategy was sometimes inaugurated by "freedom day"—the day marking the transition from a mitigation to an uncontrolled transmission strategy. All governments that made an abrupt transition from controlled to uncontrolled transmission—putting faith in vaccines to protect hospitals from a deluge of Covid-19 patients—soon discovered their faith in vaccines was misplaced. While Bill Gates, Anthony Fauci, the vaccine makers, the Trump and Biden administrations, and the Boris Johnson government, promised a vaccine-delivered return to normal, one inconvenient fact was ignored: If control measures were lifted, there were enough people who couldn't or wouldn't get the vaccine that the uncontrolled circulation of the virus among this population would produce enough illness that hospitals would be overwhelmed. Indeed, lifting public health measures, despite the arrival of vaccines, would make matters worse.

To see why, imagine three scenarios. In the first, a virus, left to spread unchecked, hospitalizes one of every two people. In the second, public health measures are implemented. The result is that only one of every 10 people is hospitalized. In the third, a 100 percent effective vaccine is developed. Anyone who receives it, is protected against hospitalization.

In our third scenario, a "freedom day" is declared and all control measures are lifted. But only half the population elects to get vaccinated. What happens next? In the half of the population that accepts vaccination, everyone is protected, and no one is hospitalized. But in the other half, the virus circulates freely, unchecked by mitigation measures. Where mitigation measures once protected everyone, now half the population is completely unprotected. If one of every two is hospitalized, as we've assumed above, then 25 percent of the population as a whole ends up in the hospital (50 percent hospitalization x the unprotected 50 percent of the population = 25 percent). Hence, we've gone from a 10 percent hospitalization rate under a no vaccine-mitigation scenario (scenario 2), to a higher 25 percent rate under a "freedom day" scenario in which only half the population is vaccinated (scenario 3). Growing morbidity and mortality following a shift from mitigation to living with Covid, is precisely what happened in the United States, United Kingdom, Austria, and Israel, and in some provinces of Canada. The reason why was because many people in these countries and provinces either refused to get vaccinated or were unable to be immunized. When mitigation measures were lifted, they were left completely vulnerable.

The reality that the wide availability of vaccines will only relieve stress on hospitals and healthcare resources if a very large fraction of the population, including children, is immunized, was blithely overlooked. When public health measures were lifted, morbidity and mortality increased, rather than diminished. The outcome was predictable to anyone not enveloped by the fog of mystification produced by the vaccine champions. Still, the vaccine champions kept up their misleading patter about vaccines. Vaccines, they insisted, were the only, or best, way to end the pandemic—despite the evidence. In the meantime, China, which was also producing vaccines and inoculating its population, continued to pursue its zero-Covid strategy. Life had, long ago, returned to near normal in China. And cases and deaths remained extraordinarily low. Exactly what were the Chinese doing?

***

The best way to understand what the Chinese were doing is to understand that "China always set zero as their goal," as *The New York Times* reporters Rebecca Tan and Alicia Chen noted in the summer of 2021.[15] Beijing took Covid-elimination seriously—perhaps more seriously than any other country, with the exception of North Korea.

There was no particular genius in China's approach to stamping out Covid-19 within its borders. Beijing's strategy was based on an axiom. As author Michael Lewis explained, "One thing that is inarguably true is that if you got everyone and locked each of them in their own room and didn't let them out to talk to anyone, you would not have any disease."[16] China did not go to this extreme, but what Beijing did do, was close.

China's initial response to the outbreak was to lock down Wuhan, the city in which the disease was first identified. Only one member of each household was permitted to leave their place of residence every few days to gather provisions.[17] This was a variation on Lewis's "lock everyone into their room and don't let them out until the disease is gone" approach. Within a matter of weeks, the city's 11 million people were tested for SARS-CoV-2.[18] Sixteen temporary hospitals were rapidly built to isolate people with mild to moderate symptoms. Because patients were quarantined in a hospital and not at home, family residences did not become petri dishes for the growth and transmission of the virus. If a patient's condition worsened, they were transferred to a regular hospital. By March 10, the outbreak had been brought under control, and the temporary hospitals were no longer needed.[19] After 76 days, infections had been driven to zero, and the city was reopened.

At the same time, Beijing rapidly set up a country-wide contact tracing system,[20] eventually developing a highly stringent definition of contact. Anyone who had been in a building four days before or after a person who developed Covid-19 symptoms or tested positive for the disease was deemed a contact and quarantined.[21] While this may appear to be draconian, and a measure guaranteed to gather large numbers of people in its net, it should be remembered that case numbers were exceedingly low. The odds of falling into this broad definition of a contact were infinitesimally small. (Two years into the pandemic, less than seven one-thousandths of one percent of Chinese residents had tested positive for the disease. The odds of encountering a person who had tested positive over this period were less than the odds of being struck by lightning.)

Having eliminated the disease within its borders by severing the chains of transmission, China implemented additional measures to minimize the chances the virus would seep into the country from outside. While it didn't go as far as North Korea, which shuttered its borders completely to seal itself off from the world, Beijing did enforce tight border controls.[22] Travellers required special government approval to enter the country, and those who received visas were required to quarantine for at least two weeks after arriving,[23] and for two weeks before their arrival. Quarantine was required for all travellers, including those who were fully vaccinated.[24] These controls were not infallible. Occasionally, the virus evaded the border restrictions and slipped into the country. When it did, public health authorities acted quickly and decisively. When nine airport cleaners at the Nanjing Lukou International Airport tested positive for Covid-19 during routine testing, the city immediately imposed lockdowns and tested its 9.3 million residents in just two weeks.[25]

Zeng Guang, the former chief epidemiologist of the Chinese Center for Disease Control and Prevention, described China's strategy as one that didn't "simply treat infected patients but cut off the disease infection routes by screening out and quarantining every close contact or potential virus carrier through prompt epidemiological investigations."[26] In others words, China simply followed the tenets of epidemiology 101. As the *British Medical Journal* explained:

> China mobilised quickly and within two months had contained the epidemic and eliminated local infections in the country. There were no magic bullets in the tools it used: the methods were old school

public health strategies, which are often called non-pharmacological interventions. Other countries also successfully eliminated local infections, showing that elimination of an emerging disease with pandemic potential is possible by using non-pharmaceutical interventions alone. Public health methods such as mask wearing, hand washing, social distancing, and restriction of public events and travel played an important part. Identifying and quarantining people with covid-19 and their close contacts was also critical.[27]

China's success, then, was due, not to vaccines and new technology—the lodestones of the West's pandemic response—but to old school public health methods.

**

In an April 2021 study, the British medical journal, *The Lancet*, compared five OECD countries that pursued an elimination strategy with 32 others that opted for hospital surveillance-based mitigation. Australia, Iceland, Japan, New Zealand, and South Korea had followed China's lead, imposing tight border controls, along with test, trace, and quarantine methods, to eliminate community transmission. The study's authors compared the two groups on "COVID-19 deaths, gross domestic product (GDP) growth, and strictness of lockdown measures during the first 12 months of the pandemic."

The study found that:

- The mortality rate was 25 times lower among countries that pursued elimination.
- Lockdown measures "were less strict and of shorter duration" in the elimination group.
- "GDP growth returned to pre-pandemic levels in early 2021 in the five countries that opted for elimination, whereas growth [was] still negative for the other 32 OECD countries."

On the basis of their analysis, the authors concluded that governments that pursued the elimination strategy not only performed better at protecting the health of their citizens and saving lives, but "also better protect[ed] their economies and minimise[d] restrictions on civil liberties compared with those that strive[d] for mitigation."[28]

The New York Times noted that "In many countries, debates [had] raged over the balance between protecting public health and keeping the economy running."[29] *The Lancet* study showed that the debate was based on a false dichotomy. Protecting public health and keeping the economy running were not antithetical goals. On the contrary, the countries that performed best at protecting public health, also did best at keeping their economies running. *The New York Times* noted that in China, there was little debate. Rather than opting for public health over the economy or the economy over public health, Beijing protected both.[30] Indeed, in 2020, China's economy "was the only major world economy to grow in a year ravaged by the pandemic," observed *The Wall Street Journal*.[31] China was also one of the few countries to prioritize public health—protecting its citizens at a level commensurate with what is achievable within the limits of epidemiological best practice.

In sum, by acting quickly and decisively, with zero-Covid as its goal, China stamped out the virus within its borders, and then enacted stringent border controls to keep the virus out. Chinese citizens quickly resumed their former lives, unfettered by the recurring restrictions and prolonged lockdowns that became the bane of countries that opted for hospital surveillance-based mitigation. At a time North America and Europe were locked down, *The New York Times* would note that "China resembles what 'normal' was like in the pre-pandemic world. Restaurants are packed. Hotels are full. Long lines form outside luxury brands stores." Instead of conducting meetings on Zoom, people were meeting face to face to talk business, catch up with friends, and celebrate special occasions.[32] As *The Lancet* study found, a zero-Covid approach—the strategy China showed the world could work—outperformed the strategies favored by the United States and most of the other rich countries, and did so not only in relation to public health, but in connection with the economy and civil liberties, as well. It saved vastly more lives, minimized economic damage, and let people get back to their regular lives quickly, free from the restrictions that sparked anti-lockdown protests throughout the West.

***

New Zealand, Aotearoa as the Indigenous people call it, had been one of the bright stars in the pandemic control firmament. Emulating China's elimination strategy, Wellington had shuttered the country's borders to all but a trickle of people, mostly returning citizens, quarantining them in isolation facilities for two weeks. The approach had produced cumulative morbidity and mortality rates almost as low as China's. By early October 2021, New Zealand had experienced 922 cases per million, higher than China's 68, but much lower, by a factor of over 140, than the United States' 132,000. There had been five deaths per million residents of the country, a shade over China's three per million, and 425 times lower than the comparable figure for the United States.

What's more, by the summer of 2021, the economy had been fully reopened for a year (except for restrictions related to border closures.) Physical distancing requirements had been lifted, and no one wore masks in the streets. The strategy, an unequivocal success, was highly popular, supported by the people, and by all parties in parliament.

The border restrictions, however, were not popular with the business community. Former prime minister John Key attacked the government, accusing the prime minister, Jacinda Ardern, of turning New Zealand into what he called a North Korean-style hermit kingdom. Key, one of the wealthiest people in New Zealand, had worked for investment banker Merrill Lynch as global head of foreign exchange before entering politics, and was chairman of ANZ Bank New Zealand. He and other business leaders demanded the government reopen the country's borders for business.

In late August, 2021, an opportunity arose for corporate New Zealand to press its case. An outbreak erupted in Auckland, the country's biggest city. By global standards, the outbreak was more like a trickle. The seven-day rolling average of new confirmed cases per million was 0.03 from September 3 to September 8. At the same time, new US infections were running at over 4.6 per million—more than 150 times higher. Still, the business community seized on the outbreak. The Ardern government was pressured by the country's business-owned media to "admit" the elimination strategy had failed and that the only way forward was for the country to reopen and learn to live with Covid. Ardern caved. She announced that New Zealand would no longer be able to eliminate the virus. Instead, the country would move to hospital surveillance-based mitigation, and ramp up its vaccination program.[33]

As New Zealand turned away from its elimination strategy under business pressure, the South Korean government, which until that point had been hailed as one of the leading countries in its response to the pandemic, did the same. Seoul decided it was time to transition from an elimination strategy to what it called a "co-existence" strategy aimed at managing Covid-19 to the level of the seasonal flu—that is, treating the novel coronavirus as an endemic disease, one that can, on occasion, strain hospitals and medical resources, but doesn't normally overwhelm them. The country would let infections soar, so long as the strain on hospitals was held in check. Seoul was, thus, willing to accept a higher number of deaths than it had under its elimination strategy, in the interests of fully reopening its economy to unfettered profit-making. To protect hospitals from strain, the country would accelerate its vaccination program and stock up on antiviral medication—a move that would fill the coffers of Moderna, Pfizer, and Merck. Once the country achieved vaccination targets of 70 percent of the entire public, 80 percent of adults, and 90 percent of older adults—and then allowing two-weeks for antibody formation—Seoul would lift restrictions and return to business as normal.

To manage the demand on hospitals, the South Korean government was set to purchase 38,000 treatments of Molnupiravir, Merck's antiviral pill for treating mild to moderate cases of Covid-19. The drug hadn't yet been approved for use in the United States, but it was shown in trials to cut hospitalizations by 30 percent. It would thus prove useful to a modest degree in limiting hospitalizations once curbs were lifted on the circulation of the virus. The drug maker had set a market price of over $700 per treatment—more than 10 times its cost of production.[34]

Seoul's plan was good for business and good for the US pharmaceutical industry. Whether it was good for South Koreans, however, was another matter.

***

If Beijing set zero Covid-19 cases as its goal, Washington set protecting the stock market and avoiding disruptions to business as its goals—along with one other: developing a vaccine. From day one, "all expert talk" in the United States, "was about how to speed the production and distribution of vaccines," observed Michael Lewis. "No one seemed to be exploring the most efficient and least disruptive ways to remove people from social networks"—the method China pursued with great success and that the World Health Organization described as "proven" and "known to work." There is no difference, Lewis, wrote, "between giving a person a vaccine and removing him or her from the social network: in each case, a person [loses] the ability to infect others."[35] Yet in the United States, the vaccine was king, regarded by the official cognoscenti—the White House and its science advisers, the pharmaceutical industry, Bill Gates, and practically every mainstream journalist—as the sole route, yes, *sole* route to an exit from the pandemic. Anthony Fauci even likened a vaccine to the cavalry.[36]

Anyone who lived in North America and Western Europe—or indeed, just about anywhere in the world outside China—would very likely have heard repeatedly in the months following the viral outbreak that at some point, within a year to 18 months, a vaccine would be developed, after which it would be quickly manufactured and distributed, allowing humanity to put the pandemic behind it and all of us to resume our lives as before. What we very likely didn't hear, amid all the celebration of vaccines and how they would save us all from the inconvenience of Zoom calls, lockdowns, and masks, was that China had already largely put the pandemic behind it, even well before Russia won the vaccine race, introducing the first Covid-19 shot, aptly named Sputnik V (V for vaccine), to recall the other Sputnik, the first satellite and Russia's (or more precisely, the Soviet Union's) victory in the race to space.

Fauci, the most visible infectious disease expert in the countries that orbit the United States, (apart from Bill Gates, whose expertise was self-declared), was the septuagenarian doctor *cum* mandarin who appeared to be the voice of reason and science against the obvious nonsense of the self-declared genius, Donald Trump, a megalomaniac who wondered whether a bright light shone deep inside the body, or maybe Lysol injected into the veins, might cure Covid-19. Fauci had spent most of his career overseeing research on vaccines and therapeutics as the solution to infectious disease. Of two approaches to dealing with contagious afflictions—pharmaceutical interventions (drugs or vaccines) or non-pharmaceutical ones (testing, contact tracing, and isolation)—Fauci was clearly on the pharmaceutical side. It's no surprise, then, that the New York physician promoted vaccines as "the cavalry." But here's a question: How is it that Fauci, whose career inclined him to see solutions through the lens of pharmacy, became the go-to expert on how to beat the pandemic? And why was Bill Gates, who had spent years promoting vaccines, popping up everywhere, echoing Fauci, extolling the merits of inoculations? To be sure, *safe* and *effective* vaccines are highly desirable, responsible for saving countless millions of lives, and represent a significant advance in public health. But were vaccines the gold-standard for defeating the Covid-19 pandemic? Since the pandemic had already been defeated in some parts of the world without recourse to vaccines, and Covid-19 vaccines had, at this point, yet to be developed, the single-minded focus on vaccines to the exclusion of elimination, required explanation. Surely, any go-to expert on how to defeat the pandemic ought to have had a Chinese name.

Despite overwhelming evidence that an elimination strategy got results, the United States and its satellites laid all their bets on a cow, hardly an animal to perform well in a horse race. The cow had a Latin name, *vacca* (*vache* in French and *vaca* in Spanish), which is related to *vaccinus* (the Latin adjectival form of cow) and *variolae vaccinae*, or cowpox. The vaccine pioneer Edward Jenner had discovered that an inoculation of cowpox, a disease that is harmless to humans, provides protection against a related pathogen, smallpox. Hence, Jenner's smallpox serum, which contained the cowpox virus, was named *vaccine*, after cows. To all expert opinion in the US orbit, Jenner would no longer be renowned solely for pioneering the smallpox vaccine—he would also become the intellectual precursor of a (failed) solution to the Covid-19 pandemic.

To be sure, not *all* expert opinion was for vaccines as the solution to the pandemic. It's just that all expert opinion that mattered was. There were plenty of experts who warned that vaccination alone was not the way out of the pandemic. But no one was listening.

The WHO director-general counselled that "vaccines alone will not get any country out of this crisis"[37] and "vaccines alone cannot solve the pandemic."[38] He added that "there is no silver bullet at the moment and there might never be. For now, stopping outbreaks comes down to the basics of public health and disease control; testing, isolating and treating patients and tracing and quarantining their contacts."[39] In other words, doing what China did. Dr. Leana Wen, an emergency physician and public health professor at George Washington University, echoed Tedros. "We should not be thinking of the vaccine as a silver bullet," she warned.[40] Emer Cooke, the Executive Director of the European Medicines Agency—the body that regulates drugs in the European Union—said the same. "Vaccines alone will not be the silver bullet that will allow us to return to normal life."[41] Dr. Peter Hotez, the dean of the National School of Tropical Medicine at Baylor College of Medicine, joined the chorus. Vaccines, he said, "are not magic solutions."[42] Simon Clarke, a professor of cellular microbiology at the University of Reading observed that "There's been an attitude in some quarters that a vaccine is our automatic savior." While vaccines are "really important," he said, "they're not a silver bullet."[43] Dale Fisher, an infectious diseases specialist at the National University of Singapore warned that "There's no fairy-tale ending where we wake up and there's a vaccine that's 100 percent effective and 100 percent of people around the world can get it and take it and Covid's gone."[44] Ana Bento, an epidemiologist, warned that vaccines are not a panacea. So too did the North Korean state media—but no one in Washington ever listened to them.[45]

Exhibiting a subtlety of thought conspicuously absent among the coterie of Fauci, Gates, and their merry band of vaccine cheerleaders, Andrew Lee, an expert in global public health at the University of Sheffield, noted that the coronavirus would only go away if governments pursued a zero-Covid strategy. "If a successful vaccine is developed *and* governments adopt an elimination mind-set, the coronavirus could go away. But such an outcome would be impossible if half the world is willing to live with the virus, enabling it to settle into a pervasive flulike pattern, only deadlier" (emphasis added).[46] Summing up the view of the unheeded experts, Martin McKee, a professor of public health at the London School of Hygiene and Tropical Medicine, put it bluntly: "Anyone who says that vaccines alone can end the pandemic is wrong."[47]

And yet that's what expert opinion at the White House said. The Trump White House, champion of the vaccine strategy, announced that it was "fully focused on defeating the virus" through therapeutics and a vaccine. Ending "this virus through medicine is our top focus."[48] *The New York Times* noted that while the administration approached the pandemic in a confused, poorly coordinated, *ad hoc*, and largely apathetic way, the exception was its attention to developing a vaccine, which was methodical, concerted, and evinced a strong commitment.[49] Biden followed Trump's lead on pandemic response, as on so many other files, from China to Iran. "Vaccination is key to getting the pandemic under control and keeping the economy strong," Biden announced.[50] The availability of vaccine doses for every US American adult led the new US president to effectively declare the Covid-19 pandemic over in the summer of 2021, despite the fact that the United States continued to post among the world's worst Covid-19 morbidity and mortality figures. It was as if the White House defined the end of the pandemic as the day vaccines arrived. Campaigning for president in the autumn of 2020, Biden launched a withering attack on Trump. "Anyone who is responsible for that many deaths should not remain as president of the United States of America." At the time, 220,000 US Americans had died of Covid-19. Ten months into Biden's presidency, the death toll had climbed by a further 350,000—more than under Trump's presidency. "It would seem," editorialized *The Wall Street Journal*, "that Mr. Biden has done no better than Donald Trump in defeating Covid despite the benefit of vaccines."[51]

Relatedly, the US pharmaceutical industry chimed in with a panegyric to itself. "We led the world in responding to this pandemic," said one drug-company executive,[52] apparently unaware that China had kept the Covid-19 death toll to a miniscule fraction of the US toll per million, without the US pharmaceutical industry's "leadership."

As to major newspapers, they continued to propagate nonsense about how "Vaccines are the main weapon fighting the pandemic,"[53] which was true, in the sense that it was the only weapon left after the one that was proved able to slay the Covid-19 dragon—elimination—was rejected as too costly and a danger to the stock market.

One of the stupidest pronouncements by a journalist on the presumed power of the vaccine strategy was made by *New York Times* reporter Donald G. McNeil Jr. on November 30, 2020, the eve of the vaccine roll-out in the United States. "The United States may well become the first country to bring the virus to heel through pharmaceutical prowess," McNeil declared, with more than a touch of US boosterism.[54] On that day, 1,344 US Americans died from Covid-19 (while zero died in China). By January 12, the daily death toll had more than tripled to 4,460 (zero in China). Ten months later, on September 16, 2021, deaths were running at more than 3,000 per day (zero in China). US "vaccine prowess" had not brought the virus to heel. On the contrary, more people were dying than died before vaccines were available.

The United States would not bring the virus to heel through vaccines anymore than it would defeat, through drugs, any of its other public health problems—from obesity to type 2 diabetes, heart disease to cancer. These problems are largely the unwelcome consequences of capitalism. The food industry lards its products with fat and sugar to delight taste buds, with predictable consequences for the waistlines and arteries of consumers. Diet, exercise, weight loss, and reduced exposure to carcinogens—the solutions to these public health problems—are anti-capitalist, in the sense that they displace profit-generating pharmaceutical interventions. Likewise, the non-pharmaceutical public health measures that can bring pandemics to heel, and prevent them in the first place, are anti-capitalist too, so far as they displace therapeutics and reduce the need for vaccines. As one of the public health figures featured in Michael Lewis's book *The Premonition*, put it: "From the point of view of American culture, the trouble with disease prevention [is] that there [is] no money in it."[55] The expert had used "American culture" as a euphemism for "capitalism."

The incentive structure underlying capitalist healthcare favors drugs to manage chronic conditions rather than prevention to keep them at bay. As a result, the response to the Covid-19 threat was predictable. While China, and a handful of other countries, emphasized aggressive containment through non-pharmaceutical public health measures, most governments limited their response to managing infection levels to prevent the number of cases from exceeding hospital capacity, while awaiting a vaccine. The response was shaped, not by what was best for the health of the public, but what was best for the health of the business community. For governments enthralled to capitalist imperatives, it was far better to minimize the impact on business activity of pandemic control measures, avoid costly public health expenditures, and support profit-making opportunities in vaccine development, than to implement stringent measures, as China did, to stop the outbreak.

The WHO's assessment of the world's response to the pandemic noted that "while much of the early response to COVID-19 involve[d] missed opportunities and failure to act, there [were] some areas in which early action was taken to good effect, most notably in research and development (R&D) and, in particular, vaccine product development." This invites a question: Why did much of the world fail to incur the costs necessary "to curtail the epidemic and forestall the pandemic," but succeeded so notably in "vaccine product development"?

To answer that question, it is necessary to address four topics, which I do in the chapters to follow.

The first topic concerns who it is that made the decisions on how to respond to the pandemic (if to respond at all) and what their interests are. In most countries, governments are dominated by members of a billionaire class and by politicians indebted to them. Not only do these decision-makers make decisions with capitalist class interests in mind, they operate within a capitalist framework which limits the range of decisions that can be made without impairing the smooth functioning of capitalist economies. Even if decision-makers aren't already inclined to formulate policy to comport with capitalist class interests—and they very much are—the structure of the capitalist economy compels them to act in ways that protect and promote capitalist interests. Capitalist interests discouraged the pursuit of elimination, for its perceived injurious effects on business activity and profit accumulation, and encouraged the development of vaccines as a profit-making opportunity.

The pharmaceutical industry—central to the pandemic response of most capitalist states—is the second topic. Like the state in capitalist society, Big Pharma is dominated by wealthy investors, whose interests come first. The industry, like government, operates within a capitalist framework. All decisions must ultimately serve one aim: the profitable production of drugs. While advantages to public health may follow as a by-product of the pursuit of profit, they are by no means necessary. Enlarging the interests of the industry's capitalist owners is the industry's sole mission. As a consequence, the production of useless and even harmful drugs is tolerable, so long as profits are produced. The pharmaceutical industry, with the complicity of Washington, fast tracked the development of Covid-19 vaccines with little regard for their safety, arguing that safety protocols needed to be circumvented to address a public health emergency—one that need not have happened and was of Washington's own making.

The third topic is Bill Gates, a significant member of the US capitalist class. Gates uses his vast wealth to pursue pet projects under the guise of performing charitable works, including promoting vaccines and capitalist pharmacy as the solution to the world's most significant public health problems. Gates offers a concrete example of how members of the capitalist class use their wealth to shape political agendas to expand their own interests at the public's expense.

The final topic is Operation Warp Speed, Washington's Covid-19 vaccine program, which used public money, and capitalized on publicly-funded research, to develop vaccines and therapeutics in record time. Washington transferred these publicly developed goods to the private sector for private commercial gain. Many decision-makers and influencers in Washington had stakes in the vaccine makers that profited from this transfer. Firms such as Pfizer, Moderna, and AstraZeneca made a killing, thanks to billions of dollars in publicly-funded research and advance purchase orders from governments. The model of "socialism for the rich"—taking money out of the pockets of taxpayers and putting it into the pockets of private enterprise—is the basis, not only for capitalist pharmacy, but for capitalist economics as a whole.

CHAPTER 3

THE CAPITALISTS' STATE

*In the United States, tycoons and business
executives ... exercise enormous sway among
politicians of both parties.* — The New York Times[1]

*The Fortune 500 and the US Chamber of Commerce
didn't just influence, they made policy.*
— Veteran trade analyst Alan Tonelson[2]

In his 2020 book *The System*, former Clinton labor secretary Robert B. Reich argues that "A powerful money-fueled oligarchy has ... the lobbying and campaign-financing muscle to mold the rules in their own favor. They can win enormous tax cuts, suppress financial and environmental regulations, acquire new patents and subsidies, fight for free trade." In short, they use their wealth and influence to win a long list of contests that pit their interests against those of everyone else.[3]

Reich argues that whether US presidents come from wealthy families or not, they are surrounded by advisers, cabinet members, and members of Congress who do. "Their norms are of those who earn more than $300,000, whose kids go to private school and whose primary savings are in the stock market rather than their homes. Their assumptions are different in profound ways from most struggling Americans."[4]

Consider William M. Daley, Obama's chief of staff from 2011 to 2012. Presidential chiefs of staff wield considerable power. They control access to presidents and manage their schedules. Before stepping into his role as the president's top aide, Daley was a high-level executive at JPMorgan Chase, a global investment bank, where he made $5 million a year. He also served on the boards of Boeing, the aerospace and weapons manufacturer, and the pharmaceutical company Abbott Laboratories. Daley is a member of the Council on Foreign Relations, a business think tank associated with the Rockefellers and Chase Manhattan Bank, which brings together high-level people from business, government, media, the military, and universities to develop foreign policy recommendations. Daley wasn't the only Obama chief of staff who had a background in finance. So too did Rahm Emanuel, who worked for Wasserstein Perella. Jacob Lew, another Obama chief of staff, worked for the investment bank Citigroup. Biden's chief of staff, Ron Klain, was a partner in the law firm O'Melveny and Myers and later general counsel and executive vice president at the venture capital firm Revolution LLC, where he was paid $2 million a year. Donald T. Regan, Ronald Reagan's chief of staff, served as chairman and CEO of Merrill Lynch, at the time the largest and richest brokerage firm in the world. A famous video clip, showing Regan imperiously commanding Reagan to "speed it up," as the president spoke to the New York Stock Exchange, hinted at who was really in charge.

To show how the wealthy dominate US politics, Nicholas Carnes, a professor of public policy at Duke University, points out that if millionaires were a political party, they would have a majority in the House, a super-majority in the Senate, and a representative in the White House, even though they comprise less than three percent of families. In contrast, if blue-collar workers were a political party, they would have fewer than two percent of seats in Congress, and their party's presidential candidate would never have sat in the White House.[5] Despite its pretensions of being the world's greatest democracy, the United States is, in point of fact, a plutocracy—a country governed by the wealthy.

***

The top decision makers in the US government are often wealthy before they enter government service, and if they're not wealthy before, they become so afterward.

The United States' first president, George Washington, was the infant country's richest citizen, worth about $500 million in today's dollars. Washington owned 300 slaves and vast land holdings. His Mount Vernon estate spanned 8,000 acres, about 10 times the size of Central Park. Thomas Jefferson and James Madison were also spectacularly wealthy. Other presidents—the Roosevelts, the Bushes, Kennedy, and Trump—were born into wealthy families.

Barack Obama and Bill Clinton weren't wealthy when they were elected president, but became multimillionaires after they left office. Ambitious people with highly developed communication and leadership skills can parlay their recherché talents into handsome fortunes by diligently catering to the interests of their wealthy backers as president.

Nearly half of the members of Congress were millionaires in 2010, compared to a tiny percentage of the US population, while over 10 percent were decamillionaires. Among the richest members of Congress at the time was John Kerry, who would later make a bid for president, serve as secretary of state in the Obama administration, and become the climate czar in the Biden cabinet. He is worth over $238 million.[6]

By 2020, the number of millionaires in Congress had climbed. Now, more than half of Congress comprised people with stratospheric wealth. House Speaker Nancy Pelosi was worth $115 million, while Senate Majority Leader Mitch McConnell held assets of over $34 million.[7] Forty-nine of 535 members of Congress, almost 10 percent, were decamillionaires, having a net worth of $10 million or more, while six were centimillionaires, worth $100 million or more.

In 2021, most members of the Biden cabinet were millionaires or multimillionaires. Fifteen had assets over $1 million. Three, individually, had assets of over $35 million. Jeffrey Zients, Biden's coronavirus czar, is the wealthiest person in Biden's cabinet, with a net worth of over $90 million. He was listed in 2002 by Fortune Magazine as among the 40 richest US Americans under 40. At the time, his net worth was estimated at $200 million. Before joining the Biden administration, Zients chaired a board that advised the Obama administration—acting as what *The Wall Street Journal* called "a kind of ambassador to the business community"—earning praise from the Business Roundtable and US Chamber of Commerce. Eric Lander, Biden's science adviser, the second richest person in Biden's cabinet, was worth over $45 million. Hence, the number one and two decision-makers on the coronavirus response in the Biden cabinet were multimillionaires and the wealthiest members of the team.[8]

The Trump cabinet was no less dominated by extraordinarily wealthy people.

Trump tried to recruit Jamie Dimon, CEO of JPMorgan Chase, a giant global investment bank, as treasury secretary, but Dimon declined. Trump then turned to Steve Mnuchin. Mnuchin comes from a wealthy family. His father, Robert, a Yale graduate, was a partner of the highly influential New York investment bank, Goldman Sachs. As a youth, Steven had a red Porsche with custom plaid upholstery. Following in his father's footsteps, Steven went to Yale and became a partner at Goldman Sachs. His brother, Alan, was a vice-president. Mnuchin left Goldman Sachs to run Dune Capital, a hedge fund, and to finance Hollywood movies. While serving as treasury secretary, he lived in a $12.6-million, nine-bedroom, mansion in Washington, D.C. His net worth is in excess of $400 million.

Betsy DeVos, who served as Trump's education secretary, has a net worth of $5.1 billion, through her husband Dick DeVos, son of Amway co-founder Richard DeVos. Betsy was born to Edgar Prince, one of the wealthiest people in Michigan. Her brother Erik founded the mercenary outfit, Blackwater, now known as Academi.

Wilbur Ross, who served as Trump's commerce secretary, is worth $2.5 billion, according to *Forbes Magazine*. He purchased a $12-million mansion in Washington D.C. when he was appointed commerce secretary. He is the chairman or director of more than 100 companies. Commerce secretaries often come from wealth. Penny Pritzker, Obama's commerce secretary, is a hotel heiress (her father was one of the founders of Hyatt hotels) with a net worth of $1.85 billion. Carlos Gutierrez, who served as George W. Bush's commerce secretary, was chairman and CEO of Kellogg's, the giant agri-food company.

Gary Cohn, who served as Trump's top economic adviser, is worth $250 million. He was a long time Goldman Sachs executive. Rex Tillerson, who served for a short time as Trump's secretary of state, was CEO of Exxon. His net worth is estimated at $230 million. Trump's daughter Ivanka Trump, and her husband Jared Kushner, who acted as presidential advisers, are worth $210 million. Linda McMahon, who was one of the biggest donors to Trump's campaign, was appointed head of the Small Business Administration. She lives in a $40-million house, owns five other houses, and has a 47-foot yacht. Steve Bannon, who served for a time as Trump's chief strategist, worked at Goldman Sachs, lived in a 14-room, multimillion-dollar townhouse in Washington, and had assets between $11 million and $50 million before joining the White House. Elaine Chao, who served as transportation secretary, and her husband, then senate majority leader Mitch McConnell, have a net worth of $34 million.

Trump considered a trio of wealthy individuals to serve as commissioner of the Food and Drug Administration, the body that regulates drugs in the United States. All believed the agency's watchdog role should be reduced to relieve pharmaceutical companies of the burden of having to demonstrate that their drugs are safe and effective. The trio included: Jim O'Neill, an associate of billionaire Trump supporter Peter Thiel; Joseph Gulfo, a biopharmaceutical executive who believed regulation stifles innovation; and Scott Gottlieb, a fellow at the pro-business American Enterprise Institute think tank. Gottlieb was appointed to the position. He joined Pfizer's board—joint maker of the Pfizer-BioNTech Covid-19 vaccine—after leaving the agency.

Biden's choice to lead the agency, Robert Califf, was a consultant to a number of large pharmaceutical companies, including Johnson & Johnson, Merck, GlaxoSmithKline, AstraZeneca, Sanofi-Aventis, Bristol-Myers Squibb, and Eli Lilly. Califf, a cardiologist, is the co-founder of Duke Clinical Research Institute, a firm that runs clinical studies for pharmaceutical companies.[9] He is a vigorous proponent of collecting less clinical trial data to reduce the costs to the pharmaceutical companies[10]—an obvious advantage to the industry, but of questionable value to consumers. Forbes noted that Califf's industry ties run deep.[11]

**

A number of secretaries of state, central bank governors, and presidential economic advisers, have had careers at Goldman Sachs, one of the largest investment banks in the world. The nexus between the bank and governments is so strong, that the bank's rivals call it "Government Sachs."

Steven Mnuchin (Trump), Henry Paulson (George W. Bush), and Robert Rubin (Clinton) held senior positions at Goldman Sachs before becoming treasury secretary. Trump's chief economic adviser, Gary Cohn, already mentioned, was a 26-year veteran of the firm, ending his career at the bank as president. James Donavan, Mnuchin's deputy, worked at the bank for 25 years. Dina Powell, Trump's deputy national security advisor, was paid $1.1 million per year at Goldman Sachs before entering government service. She returned to the firm after her stint in government.

Other alumni of Goldman Sachs include: Rishi Sunak, Britain's chancellor of the exchequer (equivalent of the US secretary of the treasury); Mario Draghi, whose career included stints as governor of the Bank of Italy, chairman of the European Central Bank, and prime minister of Italy; Mark Carney, governor of the Bank of England and earlier governor of the Bank of Canada; former Italian prime minister Mario Monti; and former Australian prime minister Malcolm Turnbull.

"Government Sachs," remarked *The Wall Street Journal*, "has long seen executives move seamlessly between Washington and Wall Street."[12] The firm's connections with the US government were first established in the 1930s by Sidney Weinberg, who headed the company for 30 years, earning the sobriquet "Mr. Wall Street." A major fundraiser for Franklin D. Roosevelt, Weinberg set up the Business Advisory and Planning Council, to bring top executives together with government leaders. It was later renamed the Business Council, a "forum for top CEOs to engage in candid discourse, exchange insight and bring their uniquely informed perspective on business and industry to governmental agencies and officials," according to Goldman Sachs. The Business Council counts an assortment of billionaires and centimillionaires among its members, representing the elite of US business. Members include Amazon's Jeff Bezos, Microsoft's Satya Nadella, GlaxoSmithKline's Emma Walmsley, JPMorgan & Chase's Jamie Dimon, Pfizer's Albert Bourla, Johnson & Johnson's Alex Gorsky, and, of course, Goldman Sachs' David M. Solomon.

***

People who went to elite preparatory schools and universities are over-represented in the halls of power. In Britain, a majority of cabinet ministers, top civil servants, diplomats, and senior judges, attended patrician public schools (which would be called private schools in North America), such as Eton and Harrow, and then went on to attend Oxford or Cambridge. Members of parliament are 24 times more likely to have attended Oxford or Cambridge than members of the general public, and 33 times more likely to have gone to an elite public school. Newspaper columnists—shapers of public opinion—are vastly more likely than the general public to have attended public schools and universities catering to inherited wealth.[13]

David Cameron, who served as British prime minister, is emblematic of the kind of people who serve in the top positions in the British state. Cameron was born into a wealthy family. He was educated at Eton and Oxford. At the age of 11, he travelled from London to the United States by the supersonic commercial airliner, the Concorde, to attend the birthday party of Peter Getty, the grandson of the oil tycoon John Paul Getty. Cameron is friendly with top media and business figures, including media tycoon Rupert Murdoch, owner of *The Wall Street Journal*, among other newspapers, and socializes with the press baron's children, Elisabeth and James. Murdoch was one of Cameron's first visitors after becoming prime minister.

In the United States, house members, senators, and federal judges are far more likely than members of the general public to have attended Ivy League Schools, such as Harvard, Yale, and Princeton, training ground for America's untitled nobility.[14] Six of every 10 "of the thirty top members of the Biden team received degrees from or worked for one of the world's top ten universities," including Harvard, Yale, Stanford, Princeton, Columbia, and the University of Chicago. These universities, "all private, with massive endowments, and very expensive to attend" instill "in students the values and ideology of the ruling class."[15]

***

Before universal, one-person, one-vote suffrage, some countries practiced censitary suffrage. Censitary suffrage (*censitary* from *census*) is voting based on rank or property, where the votes of the elite are accorded more weight than those of everyone else. Today, weighting votes by wealth would be considered intolerable, but electoral systems in North America, Britain, Western Europe, and Japan, are based on a *de facto* censitary suffrage. While it's no longer true that the votes of a wealthy few carry more weight than those of common people, it is, however true, that the wealthier one is, the more power one has to influence election outcomes.

While candidates who spend the most money on their campaigns don't always get elected, they usually do. In the 2020 US senate races, the the top-spending candidates won in nearly three-quarters of races. That was an anomaly. In every other year, the percentage was even higher.[16]

Decabillionaire Sheldon Adelson (worth $35.9 billion) spent tens of millions of dollars on Donald Trump's successful 2016 presidential bid. Trump repaid Adelson, a fervent supporter of Israel, by fulfilling the casino mogul's dearest wishes: He moved the US embassy to Jerusalem; recognized Israel's annexation of two-thirds of the Syrian province of Quneitra (which Israel renamed Golan after despoiling it in 1967 and expelling its inhabitants to make room for Jewish settlers); and released from prison Israeli spy Jonathan Pollard. Adelson spent $12 million on Newt Gingrich's election campaigns. As House Speaker, Gingrich repaid his benefactor by calling for and later backing legislation endorsing the transfer of the US embassy from Tel Aviv to Jerusalem.

Biden's biggest campaign contributors were hedge-fund investors (Donald Sussman and James Simons) and investment bankers (Blair Effron and Roger Altman)—people with plenty of money. Employees of Alphabet, Microsoft, Amazon, Apple, and Facebook, contributed $15 million in aggregate to his presidential campaign. In 2011, Pfizer executive Sally Susman raised more than $500,000 for Obama's re-election bid. Major Obama fund raisers represented top US corporations, from telecommunications to Wall Street investment banks to Big Pharma. In 2012, billionaire Michael Bloomberg spent as much as $15 million of his own money supporting candidates he believed should be elected. Billionaires Jeff Bezos, Sheldon Adelson, Tom Steyer, Richard Uihlein, and Michael Bloomberg contribute tens and sometimes hundreds of millions of dollars to election campaigns. As a consequence, they have vastly more say in election outcomes than ordinary voters.

Half the money raised to support the 2016 presidential campaigns came from only 158 families and the companies they owned and controlled. These families, noted *The New York Times*, make up a distinct class, "distant from much of America, while geographically, socially and economically intermingling among themselves." One third of the families were headed by the United States' top 400 billionaires.[17] The hedge fund billionaire Kenneth C. Griffin contributed $300,000 to the campaigns of Republican candidates, a large sum, but a pittance compared to his wealth. In 2015, Griffin's after-tax take-home pay per month was $68.5 million. His campaign contributions amounted to four-tenths of one percent of his monthly income, equivalent to about $2.17 for an average US American.

Campaign donations "come with expectations," explained *The New York Times*. "Money almost always does."[18]

***

Vast wealth not only affords billionaires outsize influence over who gets elected, it also gives them access to top government decision-makers. Stefan Selig, an investment banker who served as undersecretary of commerce during the Obama administration, notes that money "talks, so Wall Street will always have access" to top decision-makers, including the president.[19]

Stephen Schwarzman, the head of Blackstone Group, a giant global investment firm, talked by telephone regularly with Trump about economic policy and other matters. Schwarzman set up a strategic and public policy forum of top business leaders to meet regularly with the US president. Rupert Murdoch talked to Trump at least once a week. A series of top CEOs paraded through the Trump White House, including Jamie Dimon, Larry Fink, head of the global investment management firm BlackRock, Eric Schmidt, chairman and CEO of Alphabet, Tesla and SpaceX chief Elon Musk, Roy Harvey, CEO of aluminum-maker Alcoa, and Jack Welch, the former chairman and CEO of General Electric. On an average week day, at least one top corporate executive visited the White House.

In 2011, the CEOs of eight major US corporations, including Larry Fink and Bill Weldon of Johnson & Johnson, sat down with

Barack Obama to discuss the economy. Not surprisingly, they advised the president to change policy to make their companies, and themselves, wealthier. Cut regulations, they said. Make it easier for businesses to get R&D tax credits. Implement policies that will spur people to move to get jobs. And speak in a more flattering tone about Corporate USA.

When TransCanada Pipelines was seeking permission to build a pipeline from Canada to the Gulf of Mexico, it was allowed to make its case to multiple undersecretaries at the US State Department, while environmental groups were denied access to even a single US official. "Although those in office invariably deny it, the notion that access is available at a price is a well-founded reality of Washington," remarked *The New York Times*.[20]

***

Top positions in government and the state, are almost invariably pathways to the upper class.

After leaving her post as head of the US central bank, and before being appointed by Biden as treasury secretary, Janet Yellen received more than $7 million in speaking fees, mainly from financial firms, like Goldman Sachs, Citigroup, and Citadel LLC. She and her husband are estimated to hold as much as $20 million in bonds, bank accounts, and shares in 13 large companies, including Pfizer, AT&T, and ConocoPhillips.

John Baird, Canada's foreign affairs minister from 2011 to 2015, stepped into a role on mining giant Barrick Gold's international advisory board after leaving political office. He also served as a director of Canadian Pacific Railway. In 2015, Baird became an adviser to Hong Kong billionaire Richard Li, son of multibillionaire Li Ka-shing.

Michael Sabia used top positions in Canada's civil service to catapult himself into Canada's corporate elite, becoming CEO of Bell Canada Enterprises, chief executive of institutional investor Caisse de dépôt et placement du Québec, and director of MasterCard

Foundation, later returning to government as deputy minister of finance and chair of the Canada Infrastructure Bank. Sabia's boss at the privy council, Paul Tellier, who for seven years was chief of Canada's civil service, transitioned to roles in Canada's corporate upper class as CEO of the railway giant Canadian National and later CEO of Bombardier, a business jet manufacturer.

The interlocked nature of the top levels of politics and business was evidenced in the SNC-Lavalin affair, a political scandal that rocked the Justin Trudeau government in 2019. SNC-Lavalin, a large Canadian engineering and construction firm, faced criminal charges of bribery and fraud. Canada's attorney-general, Jody Wilson-Raybould, was pressured by the head of the civil service, Michael Wernick, to reach an out of court settlement with the company in lieu of a criminal trial. The chair of SNC-Lavalin, Kevin Lynch, had only a short while before left government service as Canada's chief bureaucrat, and Wernick's boss. While Wernick was pressuring Wilson-Raybould on behalf of his former supervisor, Francois-Philippe Champagne, a cabinet minister, was also having discussions with the company, offering to help SNC-Lavalin avoid criminal prosecution. Champagne knew the company's CEO, Neil Bruce, well. They had worked together at a British engineering firm. These personal ties were "a reminder," remarked the country's leading newspaper, *The Globe and Mail*, "of the tight circles that can make up the top levels of business and politics in Canada."[21]

That tight circle can be discerned in another way. Many Canadian cabinet ministers and provincial premiers use their political positions to land high-level executive jobs on Bay Street, Canada's financial center. Navdeep Bains transitioned from minister of innovation, science, and industry to vice chair of the investment banking division of the Canadian Imperial Bank of Commerce. Bains followed Lisa Raitt to the bank. She held a number of cabinet roles in the Stephen Harper government. John Manley, a deputy prime minister, chaired CIBC's board after leaving politics. TD Bank hired former New Brunswick premier and Canadian ambassador to the UN, Frank McKenna, as deputy chair, while former federal cabinet minister Rona Ambrose became deputy chair of TD's investment banking division. Former premier and federal cabinet minister Brian Tobin, and former federal cabinet ministers Ed Lumley and Scott Brison, joined BMO in high-ranking positions. *The Globe and Mail* summed up the march of politicians to top jobs in banking with the headline: "Bay Street's hottest hires are former politicians."[22] Many politicians are keen to act in the interests of wealthy business owners while in office as a means of paving their way to lucrative post-political careers in the private sector.

***

Most public policy adopted by governments originates in a select group of private organizations that were set up by the business elite to formulate public policy proposals and to communicate them to decision-makers. These organizations are funded by top corporations, whose CEOs set the organizations' directions. The organizations bring together top figures in government, the military, the media, and universities, to work on policy projects with key figures from the business world. Their reports, imbued with considerable prestige given their blue-chip status, are sent to relevant government departments as input into planning and decision-making. Their policy plans are also communicated to governments by appointment of their members to top positions in the state.

One of the top policy planning organizations in the United States is the Council on Foreign Relations (CFR), which publishes *Foreign Affairs*, sometimes called the informal journal of the US State Department. The CFR was founded after World War I by bankers, industrialists, and corporate lawyers with the objective of guiding foreign policy to protect and promote US capitalist class interests abroad. Long associated with the Rockefeller family until the 2017 death of David Rockefeller, the organization's honorary chairman, the CFR remains today under the direction of top Wall Street figures.

In the early 1990s, *The Washington Post*'s ombudsman Richard Harwood wrote a blistering attack on the CFR. Harwood called the council's members "the nearest thing we have to a ruling establishment in the United States."[23] The ombudsman pointed to an astonishing fact: Council members occupied top positions in the US government.

> The president is a member. So is his secretary of state, the deputy secretary of state, all five of the undersecretaries, several of the assistant secretaries and the department's legal adviser. The president's national security adviser and his deputy are members. The director of Central Intelligence (like all previous directors) and the chairman of the Foreign Intelligence Advisory Board are members. The secretary of defense, three undersecretaries and at least four assistant secretaries are members. The secretaries of the departments of housing and urban development, interior, health and human services and the chief White House public relations man ... are members, along with the speaker of the House and the majority leader of the Senate.

Researcher Laurence Shoup has documented the degree to which the CFR and US cabinets are interlocked.[24] By his count, 11 CFR members have served as secretary of the treasury, 11 as national security adviser, 10 as US ambassador to the United Nations, nine as secretary of state, nine as secretary of defense, and nine as CIA director.

Others include:

• Chairman of the Joint Chiefs of Staff, 4
• Head of the Federal Reserve, 4
• World Bank President, 3
• President, 2
• Vice-President, 2
• Director of National Intelligence, 2
• Director of National Security Agency, 1

Harwood also expressed concern at the number of top journalists who belonged to the elite policy planning group. "The editorial page editor, deputy editorial page editor, executive editor, managing editor, foreign editor, national affairs editor, business and financial editor" of his own paper, as well as its owner, were Council members. Other major newspapers were no less well represented at the Council. "The executive editor, managing editor and foreign editor of *The New York Times* are members," Harwood noted, "along with executives of such other large newspapers as *The Wall Street Journal* and the *Los Angeles Times*, the weekly newsmagazines, network television executives and celebrities."

Today, the ranks of the policy-planning group continue to include top figures in the US news media: Max Boot (*Washington Post*); Ethan Bronner (*New York Times*); Erin Burnett (CNN); Juju Chang (ABC News); Thomas Friedman (*New York Times*); Lulu Garcia-Navarro (NPR); Bianna Golodryga (CNN); Katrina vanden Heuvel (*The Nation*); David Ignatius (*Washington Post*); Joseph Kahn (*New York Times*); Joe Klein (*Time*); Nicholas D. Kristof (ex-*New York Times*); Paul Krugman (*New York Times*); Jim Lehrer (PBS); Judith Miller (ex-*New York Times*); Terry Moran (ABC News); Bill Moyers (PBS); Rupert Murdoch (owner of *The Wall Street Journal* and Fox News); Kitty Pilgrim (CNN); Walter Pincus (ex-*Washington Post*); Dan Rather (ex-CBS News); Liz Rosenberg (*Boston Globe*); David E. Sanger (*New York Times*); Diane Sawyer (ABC News); Eric P. Schmitt (*New York Times*); Amity Shlaes (*Bloomberg News*); Robert Silvers (*New York Review of Books*); Lesley Stahl (CBS News); Jake Tapper (CNN); Dina Temple-Raston (NPR); Barbara Walters (ABC News); Vicky Ward (CNN); Leana S. Wen (CNN); Bob Woodroff (ABC News); Judy Woodruff (PBS); Paula Zahn (Investigation Discovery Channel); and Fareed Zakaria (*Washington Post* and CNN).

"The membership of these journalists in the council," wrote Harwood, "is an acknowledgment of their active and important role in public affairs and of their ascension into the [US] ruling class. They do not merely analyze and interpret foreign policy for the United States; they help make it." They are "journalists of the ruling class," as Harwood termed them. Hence, the top jobs in the

US government and news media are filled by people who belong to a Wall Street-financed and -guided organization whose purpose is to provide a mechanism by which the business elite can engineer US foreign policy.

While the Trump administration was not interlocked with the Council, the Biden administration is. In 2021, fifteen of 31 members of the Biden team were CFR members: Antony Blinken, state; Lloyd Austin, defense; Linda Thomas-Greenfield, UN ambassador; Jake Sullivan, national security advisor; William J. Burns, CIA; Kurt M. Campbell, Indo-Pacific czar; Janet Yellen, treasury; Gina Raimondo, commerce; Cecilia Rouse, council of economic advisors; Alejandro Mayorkas, homeland security; John Kerry, climate; Susan Rice, domestic council; Thomas Vilsack, agriculture; Eric S. Lander, science and technology; Jeffrey Zients, counselor to the president.

Biden foreshadowed his foreign and domestic policy in the March/April 2019 issue of *Foreign Affairs*, nine months before taking office as president. In the article, titled, "Why America Must Lead Again," Biden outlined his administration's priorities: rallying US satellites to get tough on China and doubling down on US industrial planning by significantly increasing public investments in research and development, while making "enormous investments in our infrastructure—broadband, highways, rail, the energy grid, smart cities—and in education"—with the aim of meeting "the challenge" of China to US economic and technological supremacy. Biden's policy fittingly comported with the interests of Corporate USA. Publicly-funded R&D would deliver commercially attractive innovations to US businesses, at taxpayer expense. New technologies, pumped out of publicly-funded universities and government labs, would mint new billionaires, and add to the wealth of existing ones. Corporate USA would grow fat on state-funded construction projects on broadband, highways, rail, energy, and smart cities.

On top of placing its members in key state positions, the Council also directly influences policy by dominating external advisory boards established to counsel the secretaries of state and defense and the director of the CIA. The Foreign Affairs Policy Board acts "to provide the Secretary of State, the Deputy Secretaries of State, and the Director of Policy Planning with independent, informed advice and opinion concerning matters of US foreign policy." It consists of 20 advisers, most of whom belong to the Council as members. The Defense Policy Board provides "the Secretary of Defense, Deputy Secretary of Defense and the Under Secretary of Defense for Policy with independent, informed advice and opinion concerning major matters of defense policy." The Council is well represented among its members. As CIA director, Leon Panetta announced the establishment of an external advisory board of "distinguished men and women" who would visit CIA headquarters "periodically and offer their views on managing [the CIA] and its relationships with key customers, partners, and the public." Ten of the 14 advisers Panetta named to the board—the majority—were CFR members.

"We get a lot of advice from the Council [about] what we should be doing and how we should think about the future,"[25] remarked Hillary Clinton, when she was secretary of state. Both her husband Bill, and daughter Chelsea, are CFR members, as are her immediate predecessor and successor as secretary of state, Condoleezza Rice and John Kerry, respectively.

***

To develop and assert policy preferences on domestic matters, Corporate USA works through the Business Council and the Business Roundtable.

The Business Council was established in the 1930s as a group of top business figures who act as an informal advisory council to the government. They have regular discussions with top government figures, in relaxed, informal, settings. Discussions alternate with social events, paid for by the business leaders. Today, the Business Council comprises 200 CEOs of the United States' leading multinational corporations. They hold three meetings every year with top government figures, which involve panels, interviews, and presentations, mixed with social events. Members include the chairs or chief executive officers of Microsoft, Amazon, Northrop Grumman, JPMorgan & Chase, and Goldman Sachs, along with pharmaceutical companies Pfizer, Johnson & Johnson, and GlaxoSmithKline. The Business Council's core view is that government cannot operate effectively without the "expert" counsel of the country's top business leaders.

The Business Roundtable is the policy planning extension of the Business Council. Larger than the Business Council, it comprises CEOs representing the United States' largest corporations. Its members include the chief executive officers of Amazon, Apple, AT&T, Chevron, Citigroup, ConocoPhillips, Dell, Delta Airlines, Exxon, FedEx, Ford, Fox, General Dynamics, General Motors, Goldman Sachs, IBM, Intel, JPMorgan Chase, Mastercard, Microsoft, Northrop Grumman, Raytheon, and Visa, among others. It also includes the leading executives from the pharmaceutical industry: the CEOs of Abbott Laboratories, Bristol-Myers Squibb, Eli Lilly, Johnson & Johnson, and Pfizer.

The Business Roundtable bills itself as a group of "thought leaders, advocating for policy solutions that foster US economic growth and competitiveness." Despite its professed devotion to public service, the group's sole aim is to enlarge its members' pharaonic wealth and that of the shareholders they represent. The only policy solutions they offer, are self-interested proposals aimed at expanding shareholder value at the expense of their employees and customers.

***

Top business leaders and the corporate leviathans they manage are intimately involved in financing and guiding the operations of a multitude of other policy planning groups, informally known as think tanks.

"Think tanks," a *New York Times* investigation found, are corporate lobbyists that pose as neutral researchers, "pushing agendas important to corporate donors" and acting as "vehicles for corporate influence and branding campaigns."[26] Think tanks complement corporate lobbying efforts by producing research that supports their donors' predefined public policy goals. Research findings are discussed with current and potential donors in advance, and are shared with donors before publication. Donors' views are solicited to help shape the contents of final reports. In effect, think tanks are researchers for hire, producing whatever conclusions their corporate donors pre-specify. The arrangement works well for Corporate USA. The subterfuge allows it to shape opinion by hiding its self-interested agenda behind a cloak of neutrality. "A report authored by an academic is going to have more credibility in the eyes of a regulator who is reading it," observed former FCC commissioner Michael J. Copps.[27] Think tanks work to build credibility where none exists. At the same time, as registered charities, they allow corporations to write off their public relations expenses as charitable donations.

The following examples illustrate how corporations use think tanks to promote their agendas.

Fed Ex had been pressing Congress to reduce trans-Atlantic tariffs and to allow more duty-free shipments. The logistics company worked with the Atlantic Council, a think tank that specializes in international affairs, to produce research that echoed the company's lobbying line. The Atlantic Council happily complied, pumping out a nominally neutral report to back up Fed Ex's position.

Drone manufacturers General Atomics, Boeing, and Lockheed Martin teamed up with the Center for Strategic and International Studies to produce research recommending the Obama administration change its drone policy to allow sales to other countries. The research would be published by CSIS, with no acknowledgement that the research was, in fact, a drone industry effort with a pre-set conclusion. With a report in hand echoing the industry's position, General Atomics forwarded the research to officials at the Department of Defense, including the deputy assistant secretary of state for defense trade controls. The company also sent the report to Congressional staff. A year later, the Obama administration changed its policy.

Dr. Mark B. McClellan, a Johnson & Johnson board member, led a healthcare study at the Brookings Institution, as a senior fellow. The study defended an expensive treatment for hepatitis C, costing $66,000 for a 12-week treatment. The treatment happened to be manufactured and marketed by Johnson & Johnson. At the time, McClellan was receiving $265,000 per year from the pharmaceutical company for sitting on its board, on top of his salary of $353,145 from Brookings. Presenting himself as a neutral think tank scholar, McClellan argued that "even though these drugs were very expensive, they were worth it given the improvement in a patient's quality of life."[28]

In principle, anyone can hire a think tank to create the illusion that one's agenda is supported by an independent body of neutral researchers, but only businesses have the wherewithal to sponsor this legerdemain.

***

There were 11,524 registered lobbyists in Washington in 2021, 26 for every member of Congress. Over 6,400 lobbyists work in Ottawa, 19 for every member of parliament. Most lobbyists represent large corporations or business associations. Business lobbyists span individual businesses to industries to business segments to all businesses together. Lobbyists work full time at all levels of government to persuade regulators, legislators, and executive bodies to adopt business's policy preferences. Lobbyists representing mass groups and average individuals do exist, but they are vastly outnumbered and outspent by lobbyists representing business interests.

In 2018, Australian prime minister Malcolm Turnbull bent to public opinion by proposing measures to reduce carbon emissions. According to polls, a majority of Australians believed steps should be immediately taken to address global warming, even if significant costs were involved. Turnbull's government prepared a modest initiative, but soon backed away after the coal industry pushed back. Operating through its lobby group, the Minerals Council, Rio Tinto and other leading mining companies spent $5 million lobbying legislators to drop the proposal, an effort that included hosting luxury events for senior politicians. "Their businesses bring in more money than just about any others in Australia," noted *The New York Times*, "and they tend to wildly outspend any group that challenges them politically."[29] Environmental pressure groups, including Greenpeace and the World Wildlife Fund, did their best to pressure politicians to stick to their guns. But, relying largely on funding from average citizens, they lacked the financial muscle to compete with the richly endowed mining giants. Combined, the mass-based environmental groups mustered a meager $200,000 for their campaign to support the proposal, a mere four percent of what the coal industry easily assembled to kill it.

In 2018, Amazon spent $13 million on lobbying, joining Google and AT&T, which spent slightly more, as the top lobbyists in Washington. Amazon employed close to 100 lobbyists to work with politicians on formulating policy, legislation and regulations to benefit Amazon on taxes, trade, government procurement, drones, music licensing, and other matters.

***

Businesses hire public relations firms to burnish their reputations and to mold public opinion to their point of view. The expertise and influence of public relations firms is beyond the means of average citizens and mass-based pressure groups, but all businesses of a certain size employ public relations specialists, both in-house and outsourced, to promote their agendas. Bill Gates, for example, has spent billions of dollars on public relations, allowing himself to successfully renovate his reputation as a modern-day robber baron who used monopoly pricing to rip off consumers, to a saint-like figure who selflessly doles out billions of dollars in charitable contributions from his vast fortune. It has also allowed Gates, a man without any background in medicine, epidemiology, public health, virology, or vaccinology, to present himself as an expert on vaccines, global public health, and pandemic preparedness.

Mass news media, a major source of our political attitudes and understanding of the world, are owned by large corporations and wealthy individuals. *The Wall Street Journal, The New York Post,* Fox News, and a host of other media properties, are owned by the multibillionaire Rupert Murdoch. Murdoch is well connected politically, and enjoys ready access to presidents and prime ministers. The media tycoon was close to British prime minister Margaret Thatcher and was effectively a member of Tony Blair's cabinet, according to Lance Price, a former Blair spokesman.[30] Political leaders are willing to grant Murdoch audiences, because they need to curry favor with him to avoid unfavorable coverage in Murdoch-owned media—coverage which could undermine their political careers.

The multibillionaire Carlos Slim, at times ranked as the richest man in the world, is the second largest shareholder in the New York Times Company.[31] Meanwhile, one of the world's richest people, Amazon's Jeff Bezos, owns *The Washington Post*. He spent $250 million—accumulated from the labor of over a million poorly paid, over-worked, non-unionized, robustly exploited Amazon employees—to buy the newspaper in 2013, a project that helps him shape public opinion in directions that favor Amazon specifically and his fellow billionaires as a class generally.

Owning major news media allows wealthy individuals and businesses to shape public opinion to comport with their political preferences. In this way, they are able to participate in politics at a level far beyond the capabilities of average citizens and mass-based interest groups. Billionaire Ukrainian banker Ihor Kolomoisky likened ownership of news media to "having a party in parliament," with the exception that it offered even more influence.[32]

Major news corporations are interlocked with other large businesses. For example, the media watchdog FAIR (Fairness and Accuracy in Reporting) found that six of nine media corporations had directors who sat on the boards of at least one pharmaceutical company, including Eli Lilly, Merck, and Novartis. FAIR noted that news corporations, through their reporting, were in a position to poison public opinion against single-payer health insurance, a position that would help the pharmaceutical companies with which they are interlocked.[33] Similarly, reporting that presented vaccines as the sole exit strategy from the Covid-19 pandemic would also strengthen Big Pharma's interests.

News media also depend, in part, on the advertising revenue that other businesses provide, including advertising from large pharmaceutical companies. They must not produce content that will offend their clients if they are to retain their business.

Mass news media are thus triply committed—through their ownership; via the necessity of catering to other businesses as advertising clients; and by way of interlocks with other corporations—to a point of view that is congenial with business interests and the capitalist system.

Editors and journalists perceive themselves as fair and unbiased, but—having been enculturated in capitalist societies, and often belonging to the upper class themselves—are instilled with capitalist values through their family experience, education, class background, and exposure to the mass media during their formative years. They carry inside themselves a capitalist common sense—that is, a point of view that reflects capitalist biases and values. For example, in 2018, *New York Times* editorial page editor James Bennet told his staff, "I think we are pro-capitalism. *The New York Times* is in favor of capitalism because it has been the greatest engine of, it's been the greatest anti-poverty program and engine of progress that we've seen."[34] Bennet attended Yale. His father was a high-level State Department official and university president. His brother is a US senator. Is it any wonder that Bennet, a member of the capitalist class, employed by a newspaper owned by capitalists, including one of the richest in the world, should endorse a pro-capitalist editorial stance?

What's more, the few journalists who have a radical perspective are very likely to be denied employment in major news organizations, unless they conceal their perspective. It would be difficult to imagine *The New York Times*, CNN, or Fox News, hiring avowed Marxists, and allowing them to report from a Marxist perspective. Occasionally, major news outlets do employ token leftists, in order to foster the impression that they air the views of all sides, and to challenge the notion that mass news media are vectors for the propagation of ruling class views. But the exceptions do not negate the norm. Moreover, the acceptable left boundary of political discussion in major news media is mild social democracy. It's permissible to argue that billionaires have too much power and that their influence should be reined in, but it's unacceptable to say they should be eliminated as a class.

Journalists are more likely than the average members of the public to have studied at elite schools, an indication they come from wealthy families connected to business interests, or, if not, that they have been molded to the ruling class values these schools instill. Half of *The Wall Street Journal*'s editors and writers, and over 40 percent of *The New York Times*', went to elite (top 10) universities, while 20 percent attended Ivy League Schools, such as Harvard, Yale, or Princeton, training ground for America's untitled nobility.[35]

Judith Miller, who was a top reporter at *The New York Times*, illustrates the mass media's connection to elite institutions. The daughter of a nightclub and casino owner, Miller was educated at Barnard College, a private women's liberal arts college in New York City that is now part of Columbia University. After graduating from Barnard, she went to Princeton, where she earned a master's degree in public affairs. As a reporter for *The New York Times*, she was invited to join the Council on Foreign Relations, where she networked with top figures in business, government, the military, and academe. Her career at the *Times* came to an ignominious end when the newspaper forced her to resign after she uncritically reported the pretext contrived by the George W. Bush White House for the 2003 invasion of Iraq. The ruling class journalist, to invoke *Washington Post* ombudsman Richard Harwood's appellation, defended her reporting, arguing that her role wasn't to assess the contrived intelligence Bush operatives gave her, but merely to transmit it unfiltered to the public.

Another ruling class journalist, David Ignatius of *The Washington Post*, shared Miller's view of journalism as stenography for government officials. "Personally, I don't much care if the US reports about weapons of mass destruction prove to be imaginary," he said. "Toppling Hussein's regime was still right."[36] Ignatius was born into a wealthy family. His father was president of *The Washington Post*, and held various high-level positions in the US Department of Defense. David's brother, Adi, is the editor of the *Harvard Business Review*. Both David and Adi are members of the Council on Foreign Relations. David attended Harvard University. He is a member of the Trilateral Commission, a David Rockefeller-founded body, which brings together top business, political, and academic figures to coordinate public policy among North America, Western Europe, and Japan. In 2021, the heads of the organization were a US undersecretary of defense, a former head of the European Central Bank, and the chairman of a pharmaceutical company.

The New York Times' David E. Sanger can also be counted among ruling class journalists. A graduate of Harvard University, Sanger's grandfather was a radio station owner and his grandmother was the grandniece of Elkan Naumburg, a wealthy New York City banker. Sanger "has a nickname going back at least to the 1990s of 'Scoop Sanger' from his success in publishing journalistic scoops deriving from his role as a mouthpiece for elements in the intelligence community," according to the scholar Tim Beal.[37] Sanger is a member of the Council on Foreign Relations and the Aspen Strategy Group. The latter is a US ruling class think tank, interlocked with the CFR, which brings together top US business leaders with current and former policy makers, as well as high level journalists and academics, to propose solutions to US foreign policy challenges.

CNN primary anchor Anderson Cooper is a dyed-in-the-wool ruling class journalist. He is a scion of the Vanderbilt fortune, accumulated by his great-great-great grandfather, Cornelius Vanderbilt, a shipping and railroad magnate. The Vanderbilt family is considered one of the wealthiest of all time, in the same class as the Rockefellers, Carnegies, Fords, and Astors. Gloria Vanderbilt, the fashion designer and Cornelius's great-great granddaughter, was Cooper's mother. The CNN anchor attended Yale, and spent his summer vacations working at the CIA.

FAIR illustrated the class bias in news media reporting—a bias one would expect given the nature of news corporations as businesses, and the class backgrounds of their editors and writers—by showing that in the hands of mass news media the term "class warfare" is typically used to denote a one-way struggle, that of the bottom against the top. Examining the use of "the terms 'class war,' 'class warfare' and 'class warrior' by *The New York Times*, *Washington Times*, Fox News and CNN," FAIR found that in nearly two-thirds of cases, the terms referred to bottom-up struggle, typically denoted as average citizens trying to deprive the rich of their wealth, and in only three percent of the cases did they refer to top-down struggle as capitalists exploiting their employees and gouging consumers. (In almost one-third of instances the meaning was ambiguous.) "One might expect any conflict termed a 'war' to be covered as a two-way street," concluded FAIR. "Going by media coverage, it is not so much a class war as it is a class massacre, with a revolutionary rabble siphoning wealth downward (never mind how the wealth got up there in the first place)."[38]

Business-owned news media collaborate with other businesses in shaping public opinion in favor of pro-business policies by misrepresenting in news stories lobbyists, public relations specialists, and corporate officials, as pundits and independent experts. An egregious example is MSNBC's frequent use of Barry McCaffrey, a retired US Army general, to provide commentary on news stories as a "military expert." The media outlet does not acknowledge that McCaffrey sits on the board of DynCorp, a Pentagon supplier, which has a financial interest in US power projection. FAIR reported that from 2007 to 2010, "at least 75 registered lobbyists, public relations representatives and corporate officials—people paid by companies and trade groups to manage their public image and promote their financial and political interests—... appeared on MSNBC, Fox News, CNN, CNBC and Fox Business Network with no disclosure of the corporate interests that ... paid them. Many [had] been regulars on more than one of the cable networks, turning in dozens—and in some cases hundreds—of appearances."[39]

In his study "Deciding What's News," sociologist Herbert Gans argued that news is "information which is transmitted from sources to audience, with journalists ... summarizing, refining and altering what becomes available to them from sources in order to make the information suitable for their audiences."[40] Who are the sources? Government officials—that is, people who, for the most part, are indebted to a billionaire elite, along with "experts" employed by ruling class think tanks and business enterprises.

The news media have been criticized justifiably, but often for the wrong reasons. They are decried for actively distorting the news, and while this may happen from time to time, they are not so much active agents of distortion as passive agents that uncritically report the views of organizations, including governments, dominated by corporate wealth. They assemble and package press releases and the official statements of high state officials, lobbyists and corporate dominated think tanks, all of which, if not controlled by corporate wealth, are heavily influenced by it. The media, then, are the means by which the class of top business owners and managers disseminates its views on current issues.

As academic and Clinton labor secretary Robert Reich put it, the major news media are the mouthpiece of the establishment. "That's not surprising. After all, they depend on establishment corporations for advertising revenues, their reporters and columnists rely on the establishment for news and access, their top media personalities socialize with the rich and powerful and are themselves rich and powerful, and their publishers and senior executives are themselves part of the establishment."[41]

Importantly, however, major news media conceal their function as propagandists for the corporate rich. As already noted, they fail to disclose that the pundits and "experts" they feature in news stories are mere spokespeople for corporate interests. They uncritically report the lies, distortions, and half-truths of government officials, arguing, as Judith Miller did, that their role is stenography, not assessment. As a consequence, they act not as watchdogs of power, but—as political scientist Michael Parenti once put it—as lapdogs of government officials and the corporate elite. And above all, they maintain an air of Olympian objectivity, presenting themselves as balanced and neutral, when, in fact, they are constrained in a thousand ways, through the nature and interests of their capitalist owners, through their capitalist class editors, and via their capitalist advertising clients, to present a perspective that is partial to capitalism and the wealthy elite it favors.

We would accept without argument that a newspaper owned by a trade union would likely have a trade unionist as its editor, working class people as its writers, and that its reporting would be highly sympathetic to trade union and working class struggles. It would be generally supportive of working class parties and skeptical of other parties. In short, it would be class-biased, no matter what its pretensions to balance and objectivity. In the same manner, the need to cater to businesses to generate advertising revenue, along with the ownership of news media by wealthy individuals and interlocked giant corporations and with the injection of capitalist class individuals into major editorial and writing positions, guarantees that the major news media have a capitalist class bias. Hence, what major news media present as the best or only way to deal with pandemics reflects the way of dealing with global health emergencies that suits capitalist class interests best.

***

While the upper class dominates the state through the various mechanisms explored above, the state is also compelled to act by the capitalist system itself in a manner that comports with the interests of businesses and the wealthy. If politicians fail to formulate policies and laws that support the operation of the capitalist system, the capitalist economy breaks down. If the economy breaks down, either the capitalist class sponsors a fascist movement to remove the architects of the breakdown and supress its supporters, with the fascist movement then implementing policies to revive the flagging capitalist economy, or voters elect a pro-capitalist, though non-fascist, government to engineer an economic recovery, to save themselves from the pain of the economy's breakdown.

The political orientations of the people who hold high-level positions in the capitalist state are largely irrelevant. The logic of capitalism structures the policy boundaries within which policy- and decision-makers operate, forcing conservatives, liberals, social democrats, and even communists who elect to work within the capitalist system, to operate within the same narrow pro-capital-ist policy space. The prosperity and stability of a capitalist society depends on the private owners of capital accumulating sufficient profits. If they cannot generate enough profit, they cease to invest, and economic activity grinds to a halt. To maintain stability, governments must pursue policies to support the profit-making activities of their business communities. If they choose not to, their only option is to mobilize popular support to bring the economy under public ownership and control, so that investment decisions can be transferred from private hands to the public sphere, from profit-making as its goal to satisfying public needs as its end. There is no middle ground, where working-class interests can be robustly and continually expanded within a capitalist framework at the expense of the capitalist class.

The motor that sets the capitalist machine in motion is exploit-ation. The goal of business owners is to pay their employees as little as possible in order to make profits as high as possible. That is, their goal is to achieve the highest level of exploitation obtain-able, without creating social instability and interfering with the tranquil digestion of profits. This means minimizing wages and salaries, employee benefits, and tax payouts in support of social programs, to the lowest level consistent with the preservation of social order. Government policies that benefit the working class and limit exploitation—that is, measures that allow wages and salaries to rise, benefits to grow larger, and social services to increase— reduce exploitation. But in proportion as exploitation is reduced, the chances the capitalist engine will sputter and cough increases. There is, then, a limit to the degree that a government committed to working within the capitalist system can reduce the exploitation of the working class. The more it tests the limit, the more likely it will be ousted: either by disgruntled voters displeased with the down- turn in the economy engendered by pro-working class policies that attenuate business profits and discourage investment; by a military coup organized by upper class officers; by a military coup assisted by an outside power with large investments in the country that are threatened by the government's pro-working class measures; by an indigenous fascist movement prepared to introduce an overt dictatorship to create a regime of robust capitalist exploitation; or by the invasion of a foreign power whose profit-making interests have been eclipsed by the government's pro-working class policies.

Hence, governments which elect to work within a capitalist framework either support the profit-making activities of the pri- vate owners of capital, and avoid crises that can challenge their continued rule, or they pursue policies which interfere with cap- ital accumulation, and as a consequence struggle to survive. This explains why the Labour Party in the United Kingdom, Socialist parties in Western Europe, and the New Democratic Party in Canada, long ago abandoned their commitments to socialism (the elimination of working class exploitation) and have become largely indistinguishable from conservative parties in their accept- ance—indeed, their welcoming—of capitalist exploitation. It also explains why social democratic parties are overtly and unabash- edly pro-business and pro-capitalist. Additionally, it explains why some leftist governments that have rejected a revolutionary path, and tried to pursue within a capitalist framework, policies that are robustly pro-worker and hence, necessarily, anti-capitalist, failed to survive. These include the Socialist and strongly Socialist- influenced governments of Germany's interwar years; the Popular

Front government in Spain in the 1930s; and the Allende government of Chile in the 1970s, among others. They attempted to vigorously pursue pro-worker policies within a capitalist framework, when such policies are workable only within a socialist system. The moral is: governments that pursue anti-capitalist policies within a capitalist framework fall under enormous pressure to retreat from their pro-working class, anti-capitalist programs—pressure that often leads to either the betrayal of their constituency or their demise.

***

Just as capitalism structures the environment in which political decisions are made, setting limits on the art of the possible, so too does it set limits on the art of the possible in pandemic response.

When *The Washington Post*'s Marc Fisher surveyed experts on the Covid-19 endgame in the summer of 2021,[42] all ruled out as outside the bounds of acceptable action the elimination strategy successfully pursued by China, South Korea, and New Zealand, along with Vietnam and North Korea. Julie Swann, an adviser to the Centers for Disease Control and Prevention, declared "We are not New Zealand. We neither have the will nor the ability to control every case coming into the country." Swann offered no insight into why the will and ability to emulate a strategy that had worked in other countries was absent in the United States. Vaccination, and vaccination alone, lay at the heart of her view of what was possible. If "we can vaccinate most kids, we will get to a point where we no longer need masks in schools, and we'll have a return to normalcy." The other experts Fisher surveyed offered variations on this theme: Either quickly end public health restrictions and accept continuing strain on hospitals and higher than usual mortality, or gradually lift restrictions over a longer period, perhaps as many as two to three years, until sufficient population immunity has accumulated through natural infection and vaccination, and the disease recedes into the background as an endemic pathogen that only public health professionals worry about. In other words, within a capitalist framework, the only acceptable approach to exiting the pandemic had become one in which vaccines played the central role.

CHAPTER 4

THE CAPITALISTS' NANNY STATE

Governmental willingness to invest in the most uncertain phase of a fledgling sector's development underscores the fact that states do not simply regulate markets, they are the market: an indispensable pit stop on the road to commercializing a new venture. And yet, even among those who recognize the strong role played by states in creating new markets in developing regions, very few mainstream economists...appreciate the role of the state as a leading actor even in the most developed regions of the world, such as Silicon Valley. — Linsey McGoey[1]

In various ways, both obvious and obscure, the capitalist state functions to support and facilitate the business-based upper class and its accumulation of the wealth that is produced by the labor of the employees of the enterprises the upper class owns and controls. It does so by developing the human resources and skills needed by the owners and managers of business enterprises through its management of schools, education, and vocational training; by managing the size of the work force, and hence wage levels, and recruiting talent and labor from abroad, through its immigration policy; by stabilizing the capitalist system through fiscal and monetary policy; by protecting and promoting trade and foreign investment through military and foreign policy; by creating markets for private enterprise through government procurement; by expanding the domestic market through immigration policy and integrating foreign markets through trade and investment agreements; by arranging for the overthrow of governments that resist the integration of their markets into the cosmopolitan economy; and by funding government laboratories and university researchers to produce a steady stream of innovations that can be commercialized by the corporate class. The function of the capitalist state, then, is to create the conditions for the country's capitalists to accumulate profits at home and abroad.

In the January/February 2020 edition of *Foreign Affairs*, Nobel Prize-winning economist Joseph Stiglitz and two co-authors set out to remind the US ruling class that capitalism cannot flourish without the help of the state.[2] "The invisible hand of the market [depends] on the heavier hand of the state," they wrote. The scholars pointed out that the state builds the basic economic infrastructure of roads, ports and more, without which capitalism—and ruling class wealth and privilege—would not be possible. It also finances "the basic research that is the wellspring of all progress," and staffs "the bureaucracies that keep societies and economies in motion. No successful market," they wrote, "can survive without the underpinnings of a strong, functioning state." Stiglitz *et al* thought this needed to be pointed out afresh because the US state was being weakened by tax-avoiding corporations and billionaires who were failing to furnish the state with the tax revenue it needed to defend and promote their interests. It was time for Corporate USA to step up, they warned, for by "eating up the state, capitalism eats itself." By placing the burden of funding its state apparatus upon the shoulders of the employee class—whose ability to bear the load was under growing strain—the capitalist class was digging its own grave. This was an acknowledgement that the state in capitalist society is very much a nanny state—a nanny state, not for the working class, but for the corporate class that dominates it. It is the instrument of that class.

To be sure, under the pressure of socialist and labor movements, and later in response to competition from the Soviet Union, the United States and other major capitalist states developed an array of welfare state measures—that is, a nanny state for the public. Nanny state measures acted as a prophylaxis against working class agitation that threatened to disrupt the tranquil digestion of profits, and reduced the chance of revolution. Over time, however, as the welfare state expanded, the capitalist system's ability to support generous measures for the bulk of the population was tested, especially as people began to demand more of the state. The rate of profit narrowed as the degree of exploitation was reduced through growing unionization, expanding social welfare measures, and rising working class power, with the inevitable consequence that the capitalist economic engine began to misfire. This was no more welcome by the working class than by its capitalist bosses. For workers, a weak capitalist economy means joblessness or, if not unemployment, the incessant threat of it and unceasing insecurity.

To re-orient people's expectations away from the idea that the state would continue to allow exploitation to be actively attenuated, the billionaire class promoted a neo-liberal theory that advocated the insulation of the capitalist economy from mechanisms of working-class influence. Central banks were divorced from parliaments and legislatures, and hence from the possibility of voter influence, while economic decision-making was vested in extra-parliamentary bodies, outside the influence of the working-class electorate. Businesses and the wealthy were unburdened of tax obligations, so they could invest their freed-up capital in "job creation" (or so the fable went). At the same time, the Soviet Union—which had offered a model of an alternative socialist future and so acted as an ideological rival for the allegiance of workers—dissolved, the victim of its leadership's disastrous flirtation with markets. Persuaded that market mechanisms would reverse slowing economic growth, Soviet leader Mikhail Gorbachev had embarked on a path that very quickly led to the dissolution of the first workers' state. This redounded to the capitalist class's efforts to weaken working-class influence, and to return economic policy to a path more suitable to capitalist interests.

Gorbachev faced a problem. During the years the Soviet economy was publicly owned and centrally planned (with the exception of the war years), it had grown unremittingly, providing full employment, inexpensive housing and transportation, free healthcare and education, and a host of other working-class benefits, without recessions or inflation. But the economy was no longer growing as fast as it once did. Soviet leaders had pledged to reach communism—a state of high material development, where goods and services would be so plentiful, they could be distributed according to need, rather than income. With slowing rates of economic growth after the mid-1970s, communism looked a long way off. What's more, Soviet GDP per capita continued to lag that of the United States, and was not on track to overtake it. In fact, the United States was maintaining a steady lead. That pushed the Soviet leadership into an increasingly untenable position. How could it justify socialism to its citizens, much less inspire workers around the world, when standards of living were higher in North America, Western Europe, and Japan?

It didn't help Moscow's case either, that in an effort to compete with the Soviet Union, the governments of the capitalist industrial world had created their own welfare states. Workers in the industrial West seemed to enjoy better lives than their counterparts in the socialist bloc—the states that were consciously organized to serve worker interests. In Gorbachev's view, the only way out of the dilemma was to emulate the competition. Perhaps greater openness, and a restructuring of the economy to emphasize markets, would kick the Soviet economic engine into higher gear. As it turned out, "restructuring" and "openness" produced an effect opposite to the one intended: rather than stimulating growth, pro-market policies drove the state into an economic abyss. Soon after, the union dissolved.

The story of how Gorbachev unintentionally plunged the Soviet economy into chaos has since been retold as a capitalist fairy tale. The reality is that the Soviet Union's economy was not in crisis. It had not collapsed. It had not stagnated. It was growing—at a slow pace to be sure—but every year output reliably increased. It was Gorbachev's pro-capitalist policies—not the internal dynamics of socialism—that pushed the economy from low gear into reverse gear. But in the retelling of the story, Gorbachev's capitalist blunder never happened. Instead, we're led to believe that the Soviet economy continued along its socialist path until it collapsed under the weight of its own internal contradictions—the mirror image of the vulgar Marxist view that the capitalist economy will one day do the same. This astigmatic version of events informs a favorite anti-socialist trope: the "collapse" or "implosion" of the Soviet economy proves that socialism doesn't work. But the experience of the Soviet Union proves no such thing. What it proves is that Gorbachev's seduction by capitalist ideology destroyed an economy that, whatever its demerits, provided jobs for all, free healthcare and education, inexpensive housing and public transportation, while supporting an array of progressive policies in a number of areas, including women's rights and national liberation, that put the capitalist West to shame.

The demise of the Soviet Union proved highly beneficial to the billionaire class. Business communities sought to detach the working class from the social welfare measures that had been introduced to prevent working class militancy, but which put downward pressure on profit margins and strained the capitalist system's ability to operate efficiently on behalf of its masters. With the Soviet Union's demise now widely presented by ruling class journalists and scholars as the ineluctable consequence of the socialist organization of the Soviet economy, social welfare measures could be discredited as Soviet-like, and therefore equated to the purported cause of the Soviet Union's demise. Margaret Thatcher, Britain's neoliberal prime minister, declared that the death of the Soviet Union proved that there is no alternative to capitalism. Additionally, with the USSR's dissolution, billionaire-dominated governments no longer needed to compete against the Soviet Union for the allegiance of their working classes. They were now at liberty to scale back the welfare state with virtual impunity.

At the same time, neo-liberals crafted a fable about lean government as a desideratum, but lean referred exclusively to the workers' welfare state, which was to be put on a crash diet. The corporate welfare state—fat government for the rich—was to continue apace. Capitalist governments would become lean for the working class alone, and remain bloated for the corporate class. The multifarious ways in which governments supported, hand-held, promoted, and indulged businesses were concealed, hushed up, and obscured— often through linguistic gymnastics. For example, ever since Alfred Thayer Mahan, a US naval strategist, identified a robust blue water navy as the principal means by which the United States' capitalist class could command the markets of the world, Washington had plowed taxpayer money into the building of giant fleets. The principal beneficiaries were the captains of industry and high lords of finance, whose fortunes could not have been accumulated had the US Navy not opened the markets of reluctant foreign powers, and kept them open, while at the same time protecting US commercial shipping from the navies of hostile rivals. Who paid for the US Navy's leviathans? The US taxpayer. And yet, the US military—as bloated an expression of the state as has ever existed—is rarely ever portrayed as an instrument of Corporate USA, but is, misleadingly, talked of as an instrument of "national security." This ought to prompt the question: National security for whom?

The idea that the US military exists to safeguard the security of US Americans, and not to protect the profit-making interests of a tiny sliver of the wealthiest US Americans at the top, is rarely, if ever, examined in the corporate-owned news media. That's not surprising, for the reasons we've already explored: the mass media are owned by corporations and wealthy individuals, and staffed by people from wealthy backgrounds who attended elite universities and belong to billionaire-funded and -directed public policy formation organizations. They seek out the tendentious analyses of lobbyists and public relations specialists in the pay of large corporations who they mendaciously present as impartial "experts" and "pundits." Small wonder the mass news media prefer to say little about how average citizens are paying a king's ransom through their taxes to fund what one Marine General, Smedley Butler, the most highly decorated Marine of his day, called an organization of "high class muscle [men and women] for Big Business, for Wall Street and the bankers... gangster[s] for capitalism."[3] That's not to say that the true character of the US military is a secret, to be jealously guarded and never uttered. Indeed, *New York Times* columnist Thomas Friedman, a CFR member, once famously observed publicly that "The hidden hand of the market will never work without the hidden fist—McDonald's cannot flourish without McDonnell Douglas, the designer of the F-15. And the hidden fist that keeps the world safe for Silicon Valley's technologies is called the United States Army, Air Force, Navy and Marine Corps."[4] Friedman notwithstanding, the US military is rarely called Corporate USA's fist, as much as the appellation fits.

Annual funding for Corporate USA's fist, or what historian Arno J. Mayer once called the *ultima ratio regnum* (the violence behind the rule) of capitalist globalization,[5] is immense. US taxpayers shell out more on the military than do the citizens of at least the next 12 nations combined, and as much as the next 42, depending on how US military expenditure is counted. The Pentagon's budget exceeds the combined GDP of 185 countries.[6] And the United States maintains several hundred major military bases in scores of countries abroad. Is the national security threat to the United States so great that Washington needs to lavish its citizens' tax revenue on a globe-girding military empire that casts its opponents' military capabilities into shadow?

In 2021, the world's next largest military, China, planned to spend about $200 billion on its military,[7] 83 percent less than the $1.2 trillion the United States spent when all defense spending, including that hidden in non-Defense Department budgets, was tallied.[8] China has no way of meaningfully projecting power to threaten the continental United States, and is surrounded by US military bases and US troops. The Pentagon stations 50,000 troops in Japan and 27,000 in South Korea. The United States also has major bases located in its colonies of Guam and Northern Mariana Islands, in its *de facto* colony of Marshall Islands, as well as in Australia and Singapore. US ally South Korea has 550,000 active troops, and nearly three million in reserve, which, in a time of war, would be mobilized under the command of a US general. Interoperable with the US military, the South Korea armed forces are a *de facto* US military. The US military dominates the first island chain, the string of islands that separate China from the Pacific and Indian Oceans, and controls the Strait of Malacca, the route through which China—the world's largest consumer of oil—imports its vital West Asian petroleum supplies. With its command of major shipping routes and geostrategic chokepoints, the United States is in a position to shut down maritime traffic in and out of China. The East Asian country poses no threat of significance to US national security. On the contrary, the United States poses a serious threat to China.

The next largest military is that of Russia. The country has a military budget only one-tenth as large of that of the United States, and its naval and air capabilities fall well short of those of the United States. Russia has only one aircraft carrier, which, as of 2021, was *hors de combat*. The United States, by contrast, has 20 aircraft carriers. Aircraft carriers are weapons of aggression, intended for power projection—that is, imposing their possessor's will on other countries. Russia's military, in contrast to that of the United States, is designed for self-defense, not power projection.[9] What's more, Russia faces a formidable military competitor in the European Union. The European Union's population and military budget are approximately three times greater than Russia's. France alone has a military budget as large as Russia's, and has an independent nuclear weapons force.[10] What's more, the United States has a military presence in Europe, in proximity to Russia's western borders. The Pentagon stations 35,000 troops in Germany. It also has 11,000 troops in Italy and 9,000 in Britain, along with 2,000 in Turkey. Additionally, the US Sixth Fleet commands the waters of the Mediterranean, and controls the Bosporus, the chokepoint between the Mediterranean and Black Seas. This gives Washington the capability to block Russian commercial shipping from exiting and entering the Black Sea, *en route* to and from Russia's Black Sea ports. Major US troop concentrations and bases in Japan and South Korea, along with *de facto* US control of the South Korean military, pressure Russia militarily from the southeast. A major US air base in Greenland, along with airbases in Alaska, put Russia within easy striking distance of US bombers across the Arctic circle and Bering Strait. Like China, Russia poses no security threat of significance to the United States. But the United States does present a major security threat to Russia.

North Korea (DPRK), a low-income country whose population is only one-thirteenth the size of the United States', is improbably presented as a US national security threat. The Pentagon's budget is at least 74 times greater than North Korea's, and may be up to 740 times larger. Indeed, North Korea's military spending is so insignificant, it's estimated to be roughly equal to the budget of the New York City Police Department.

North Korea's peninsular neighbor, South Korea, a virtual US colony, has a population twice the size of the DPRK's, a GDP that is many times larger, and a military budget that is 20 times greater.[11] Its military expenditures are one and a half times greater than the DPRK's entire GDP.[12] Moreover, South Korea's armed forces, as mentioned above, are a *de facto* extension of the Pentagon, organized around tens of thousands of US troops stationed on a number of bases in South Korea, including Camp Humphreys, the largest US overseas base in the world.

North Korea is incapable of attacking the continental USA except possibly by intercontinental ballistic missiles (ICBMs), which may, or may not, be capable of reaching their target. While North Korea is nuclear armed, the consensus among US national security officials is that the country's nuclear arsenal is purely defensive; a first strike against the United States would trigger a US counterstrike whose outcome would be the annihilation of the northern half of the Korean peninsula. The DPRK leadership is not mad or deranged—except in the depictions of the yellow press and Hollywood—but is coolly rational, and disinclined to act in a suicidal manner. Surrounded by US and US-allied troops to the south, in the Republic of Korea, and to the east, in Japan; in the cross hairs of US strategic missiles; and subjected to incessant harassment by US bombers, North Korea is menaced by the United States, and not the other way around. For decades North Korea has repeatedly implored Washington to sign a peace treaty, and just as often Washington has rejected the DPRK's offers.

Iran has no long-range bombers, no aircraft carriers, no naval or air bases within striking distance of the continental USA, and no long-range naval capability. Nor does it have ICBMs to strike US targets, or nuclear warheads to sit atop them. If North Korea is an insignificant national security threat to the United States, then Iran is even more insignificant. Iran's military expenditures are one sixtieth the size of those of the United States. Iran is a middle-income country with a military organized mainly for defense, and capable of operating abroad, at best, only in neighboring countries. It is continually harassed by Israel, Washington's outpost in the Middle East, whose major role in US foreign policy is to suppress countries and movements in West Asia and Northern Africa that seek to exercise independence from the United States. Iran is in no position to threaten the United States, and doesn't.

Al Qaeda and its offshoot ISIS are said to be US national security threats, and while they have been threats in the past, and may continue to be threats today, the threat posed by jihadists to the continental USA is easily defused. To remove the threat, all the United States has to do is treat others as it would have others treat itself, namely, as free to conduct its own affairs and choose its own political, economic, and cultural system, without interference and coercion from the outside. Unfortunately, the United States has, throughout its history, consistently chosen to meddle in the affairs of other countries, in order to impose on them a political and economic system that suits the purposes of US investors and exporters and exploits and oppresses the natives. The United States' incessant interference in the affairs of other peoples, no less those of West Asia, has created movements of local independence and national assertiveness whose goal has been to repel US meddling and bring an end to their exploitation by US plutocrats.

In June, 1996, al Qaeda's founder Osama bin Laden told British foreign correspondent Robert Fisk that Washington had turned Saudi Arabia into a US colony and drained its oil wealth. Despite producing more oil than any other country in the world, Saudis were burdened by high taxes and inadequate public services. The kingdom's oil wealth was used to buy weapons from US arms manufacturers that it didn't need, rather than being invested in the welfare of the Saudi population. For these reasons, he explained, the United States was "the main enemy" and Muslims should resist Western occupation of their countries, as Europeans had resisted occupation of their countries by foreign fascist forces during the Second World War.[13]

Bin Laden said that pushing "the enemy ... out of [Saudi Arabia] is a prime duty .... It is a duty of every tribe in the Arab Peninsula to fight ... to cleanse the land from these occupiers."[14] The "Americans must leave Saudi Arabia, must leave the Gulf." Washington's "attempt to take over the region" and "its support for Israel" were the causes of attacks on Western military forces in the region. The United States had turned Saudi Arabia into "an American colony."[15]

In 1998, bin Laden elaborated on why al Qaeda opposed the United States.

The call to wage war against America was made because America [is] sending tens of thousands of its troops to [the Arabian Peninsula], over and above its meddling in [Saudi] affairs and [Saudi] politics, and its support of the oppressive, corrupt and tyrannical regime that is in control. These are the reasons behind the singling out of America as a target.[16]

In May 2003, al Qaeda offered further explication of the origins of the jihadist national security threat to the United States.

The Muslim countries today are colonized. Colonialism is either direct or veiled ... masking colonialism ... is exactly what happened in Afghanistan when the United States occupied that country and installed an Afghan agent, Hamid Karzai … there is no difference between the Karzai of Yemen, the Karzai of Pakistan, the Karzai of Jordan, the Karzai of Qatar, the Karzai of Kuwait, the Karzai of Egypt, and the long list of Karzai traitors ruling the Muslim countries.[17]

In other words, West Asia's leaders are quislings who veil the indirect rule of the United States.

Continuing its treatise on the provenance of militant Islam's enmity to the United States, al Qaeda explained that:

The ruler of a country is the one that has the authority in it … the real ruler [of Saudi Arabia] is the Crusader United States. The subservience of [local] rulers is no different from the subservience of the emirs or governors of provinces to the king or the president. The rule of the agent is the rule of the one that made him agent.[18]

The jihadist organization added that:

It is important to know that the colonialist enemy might give up veiled colonialism and establish, through its armies, colonialism where there is little fear of resistance or the agent leadership could not achieve the interests of colonialism or had deviated—even in a small way—from its hegemony. For this reason, the United States chose to invade Iraq militarily, and might choose to invade any Muslim country near or far from Iraq at any time. [The United States] can occupy a country whenever it wants, and this is exactly what the United States is doing in Saudi Arabia.[19]

Commenting on the 1857 uprising of Indians against British colonialism, initiated by sepoys (Indian soldiers under British command), Karl Marx remarked that "however infamous the conduct of the sepoys, it is only the reflex, in concentrated form, of England's own conduct in India."[20] Paraphrasing Marx, it might be said that however infamous the conduct of the jihadists who attacked New York City and Washington, D.C. on September 11, 2001, it was only a reflex, in concentrated form, of the United States' own conduct in the Muslim world. No matter how strenuously one denounces al Qaeda's attack on US civilians, it remains the case that the al Qaeda rebellion against the United States would not have happened had Washington not conducted itself in West Asia in an infamous way. Had the United States allowed the people of the region to make their own political and economic choices, al Qaeda would never have arisen as a US enemy.

In short, al Qaeda is only a US national security threat because Washington has made it so. As Washington created the threat, so too can it remove it. The threat is extinguishable through a simple expedient: treating the people of West Asia and North Africa as US Americans would have themselves be treated: as free to determine their own political, economic, and cultural lives without coercion or interference.

***

If the major US national security threats are not, by any reasonable touchstone, security threats of any significance—and certainly not so great as to warrant several hundred overseas military bases in scores of countries, along with a US military budget as large as the combined budgets of at least the next twelve largest military powers—who benefits from this extravagant excess, and to what end?

Several paragraphs ago, an answer was suggested by naval strategist Alfred Thayer Mahan, *New York Times* columnist Thomas Friedman, and US Marine Corps general Smedley Butler. They defined the US military as an instrument of violence used to open foreign markets, and keep them open—gangsters working in the cause of Corporate USA. This point of view was echoed by Alexander Haig, former supreme commander of NATO and secretary of state in the Reagan administration. Haig was interviewed in 2002 by United Press International editor Arnaud Borchgrave. At the time, Washington stationed 70,000 troops in Germany, at great expense to US taxpayers. Prior to the demise of the Soviet Union, Washington had argued that US troops were stationed throughout Western Europe to deter Soviet aggression. Borchgrave wondered why US citizens were carrying a heavy tax burden to pay for a US military presence in Germany when the ostensible reason for the presence had dissolved a decade earlier.

> Haig: A lot of good reasons for that. This presence is the basis for our influence in the European region and for the cooperation of allied nations.... A lot of people forget it is also the bona fide of our economic success. The presence of US troops keeps European markets open to us. If those troops weren't there, those markets would probably be more difficult to access.

> Borchgrave: I didn't forget. I just didn't know that if the United States didn't maintain 70,000 troops in Germany, European markets might be closed to American goods and services.

> Haig: On occasion, even with our presence, we have confronted protectionism in a number of industries, such as automotive and aerospace.[21]

US troops, then, had been, and are, in Europe to deter European governments from excluding Corporate USA from European markets. Washington spends hundreds of billions of taxpayer dollars every year, not to keep US citizens safe from the threat of threat of foreign-originated violence, but to keep Corporate USA safe from the threat of foreign governments protecting their markets. The Pentagon is a massive corporate welfare program.

From Butler to Friedman to Haig and beyond, there are plenty of indications that the US military has always functioned to promote and protect the interests of the United States' wealthiest citizens—its tycoons, industrialists, and financiers. In 1907, while serving as president of Princeton University, Woodrow Wilson, the future president of the United States, delivered a series of lectures. Wilson argued that "Since trade ignores national boundaries and the manufacturer insists on having the world as a market, the flag of his nation must follow him, and the doors of the nations which are closed must be battered down." Wilson made it understood that the battering would be done by the US government—specifically, the mailed fist of its military—on behalf of the country's business community. "Concessions obtained by financiers must be safeguarded by ministers of state, even if the sovereignty of unwilling nations be outraged in the process." This might include, for example, the military occupation of a country to deter it from exercising its sovereign right to protect its own markets. Wilson added that "no useful corner of the world may be overlooked or left unused"[22]—that is, no opportunity for profit-making may be denied US exporters and investors. Wilson's secretary of state William Jennings Bryan told a business audience "that President Wilson had ... made it clear that it was official policy to 'open the doors of all the weaker countries to an invasion of American capital and enterprise.' ... Having made that point, Bryan [continued]: 'In Spanish-speaking countries ... hospitality is expressed by a phrase 'My house is your house'... I can say, not merely in courtesy—but as a fact—my Department is your department; the ambassadors, the ministers, and the consuls are all yours. It is their business to look after your interests and to guard your rights."[23] Hence, not only would the US military look after the interests of US business over-seas, battering down all doors closed to it, but the US Department of State would act as an arm of Corporate USA.

***

In his 1988 book, *The Sinews of Power: War, Money and the English State, 1688-1733*, historian John Brewer set out to solve a puzzle. How did Britain, in less than a century, grow from "a peripheral power," minor and inconsequential, into "the military *Wunderkind* of the age?" Britain's expansion, he wrote, "was impelled by the powerful forces of commercial capitalism, the desire to increase profits and accumulate wealth." But that was not all. "Great states," he continued, also "required both the economic wherewithal and the organizational means to deploy resources in the cause of national aggrandizement." Markets would need to be opened in lands where rulers opposed commercial penetration. Raw materials would need to be taken from places where the people were not pre-pared to cooperate. How were foreign lands to be opened to trade, commercial exploitation, and resource extraction? The answer was clear: via an army and navy. But troops and sailors "required money and proper organization."

"The late seventeenth and eighteenth century saw an astonishing transformation in the British government," Brewer wrote. It "was able to shoulder an ever-more ponderous burden of military commitments thanks to a radical increase in taxation, the development of public deficit finance (a national debt) on an unprecedented scale, and the growth of a sizeable public administration devoted to organizing the fiscal and military activities of the state. As a result, the state cut a substantial figure, becoming *the largest single actor in the economy* [emphasis added]."

Capitalist states remain the largest single actors in their economies today. But they act, not on behalf of the bulk of people they nominally represent, but on behalf of a capitalist class. And one important way they act on behalf of this class is by taking dollars out of people's pockets and putting soldiers in the field and sailors on the high seas to open foreign markets and keep them open.

When we think of wars, we often think of large cataclysms, involving multiple countries, and occurring on a grand scale, with visible casualties and destruction. We also think of wars as anomalies, departures from long periods of peace. As a result, we rarely think of the great powers of modern history—the United States, Britain, France, Germany, Russia, and Japan—as countries that are perpetually at war. Nor do we recognize that war is an important means by which empires are created and defended. Consider one great empire—history's largest: the United States. As anthropologist David Vine noted in his 2020 book *The United States of War: A Global History of America's Endless Conflicts, from Columbus to the Islamic State*, "war is the norm in US history. According to [Washington's] own Congressional Research Service and other sources, the US military has waged war, engaged in combat, or otherwise employed its forces aggressively in foreign lands in all but eleven years of its existence"[24]—that is, in more than 95 of every 100 years since 1776. For example, between "U.S. independence and the end of the nineteenth century, Euro-American settlers waged essentially unceasing warfare against"[25] the indigenous people of North America. It was this warfare that allowed the United States, which began as thirteen British colonies on the Atlantic coast of North America, to become a continental empire, before becoming a territorial empire with possessions in the Pacific and Caribbean. Britain's experience was the same. It fought endlessly, usually against Indigenous people who occupied land British businessmen coveted for its commercial and investment opportunities. "Military action," noted Brewer, "occurred far away, beyond the horizon: in continental Europe (where foreign soldiers fought and died on Britain's behalf), in the colonies and on the quarterdecks of British battleships. Most of the military action was out of sight."

But while much of Britain's military action, like that of the United States today, was over the horizon and out of sight, the effects were "felt on the home front, particularly on the economy." For war, "was an economic as well as a military activity: its causes"—profit-seeking—"conduct"—shaped by a country's economic resources—"and consequences"—the protection and promotion of commercial interests, were—"as much a matter of money as martial prowess." The British, concluded Brewer, viewed war as "a question of property and profit."

As "the protection afforded by the greatest of economic creatures, the state" grew, lobbies, "trade organizations, groups of merchants and financiers fought or combined with one another to take advantage of" the state's power. "They struggled for access to the corridors of power, for information that would enable them to thwart, create or affect policy," and for the support of parliamentarians who could influence "the fiscal juggernaut" to support their interests. "As their tactics grew more sophisticated, they learned to transcend their sectionalism and to appeal beyond their self-interested ranks to the public at large. By the second half of the eighteenth century some of them had learned the value of parasitism, making the state, as Adam Smith pointed out, their host if not their hostage."

The US state, as much as the British, has historically been an instrument of capitalist power, structuring, coordinating, and regulating the economy on behalf of monied interests. The US historian, William Appleman Williams, noted in his 1964 collection of essays, *The Great Evasion*, that "[US] capitalism, and more particularly entrepreneurial decision-makers of the system, has had its own tax-supported social security plan ever since the Civil War guaranteed it the opportunity and the protection to extend itself over the entire continent and outward into the world marketplace." That social security plan is the "private use of public monies." Williams noted that public subvention for private gain—the socialization of risk and privatization of its rewards—"has been, and continues to be, a central dynamic element in the success of [US] capitalism." Obfuscating this reality, the US capitalist class routinely "attributes its achievement to the creative powers of private property and individual enterprise," a fairy tale instilled into the public mind by dint of the business community's control of the mass media and its sway over public education and universities. "The competitive market economy of capitalism has not been able to sustain itself without continuing and increasing subsidy from the government—meaning taxpayers."[26]

***

China has a *dirigiste* economy. The state plays an enormous role in guiding economic activity. It does so through a planning body that sets five-year plans, recalling the planned economy of the Soviet Union; through state-owned enterprises, also recalling the Soviet Union; and through ownership stakes in otherwise privately held firms. The state also uses subsidies, tax breaks, government procurement, credit, and research and development funding, to shape economic activity and guide economic growth. "A large portion of China's economic output results from government and policy-directed investments rather than market-based forces," concluded the US secretary of defense, in his 2020 annual report to the US Congress.

While Washington prefers free enterprise to state-owned enterprises, it is not the case that the US economy is regulated by the invisible hand of the market, free from the guiding hand of the state. US investors and politicians complain bitterly about the heavy involvement of foreign states in economies abroad, while affecting to shun massive state intervention at home. But the reality is that just as the Chinese state is the largest single economic actor in the Chinese economy, so too is the US state the most consequential actor in US economic affairs. This is true today as much as it was when Alexander Hamilton articulated an industrial policy based on tariffs—a state-interventionist policy that ignited the US economic take-off. The notion that other countries practice industrial planning and the United States does not, is a myth. The US capitalist class and its intellectuals seek to portray US capitalism as relatively free from state intervention. There are two reasons for this. First, to keep the US public ignorant about its role in underwriting a state that exists to protect and enlarge the interests of a narrow stratum of billionaires. Were US taxpayers to understand that their government is an instrument of their exploitation, the legitimacy of the system would be undermined, and the US state would be destabilized. The second reason Washington conceals its massive intervention in the economy is to discourage foreign governments from doing the same. If other countries emulated the United States, they would reduce the profit-making opportunities available to US investors abroad. Washington tells other countries to do as it says it does, but actually doesn't do.

Far from the Chinese model being the antithesis of the US model, economist Mariana Mazzucato argues that Beijing has simply emulated "Washington by pouring government investment into its own versions of US government research powerhouses such as the National Institutes of Health, the Defense Advanced Research Projects Agency and the National Aeronautics and Space Administration"—public sector bodies that produce innovations for commercial exploitation by the private sector. In its industrial planning, China is doing "exactly what the US did," Mazzucato argues.

The Chinese economic model is "not communism," she contends, but is simply a recapitulation of what all great capitalist powers have done to become rich and what all rich countries continue to do to stay rich: use the state to guide economic development, relying on an array of mechanisms, including subsidies, tariffs, tax policy, import and export controls, industrial planning, publicly funded R&D, and state-owned enterprises.[27]

Mazzucato is interested in what she calls "the entrepreneurial state," the idea that the largest single economic actor of all, the state, and not the unfettered market, is the true wellspring of economic development. This view challenges the myth that bold private investors risk their capital on uncertain investments, taking chances on uncertain payoffs. On the contrary, investors are conservative, shying away from big risks. They want fairly certain returns, quickly, and aren't prepared to invest long term in ideas that may fail. Instead, they have, through their sway over the state, arranged for capitalist governments to exercise their power to take dollars out of the pockets of taxpayers and place innovations in their hands by putting scientists into universities and government labs. A host of publicly-funded laboratories and government-owned research and development agencies absorb the risk and bear the expense of producing commercially viable innovations, while allowing private investors to reap the benefits and expand their already colossal fortunes.

The following innovations were developed with public funding in government or publicly-supported university labs: commercial satellites; nuclear power; the internet; rocket technology; Google's search engine; the computer mouse; graphical user interface; GPS; the touchscreen display; SIRI and Alexa; the iPhone; quantum computing; artificial intelligence; the human genome project; magnetic resonance imaging; hybrid corn; supercomputers; and most drugs, including Covid-19 vaccines. Many were developed by DARPA, the Defense Advanced Research Projects Agency, established in 1958 alongside NASA.

Between 1971 and 2006, 77 out of *R&D Magazine*'s top 88 innovations were fully funded by the US government.[28] Writing in *The*

Guardian in 2012, Seumas Milne pointed out that the "algorithms that underpinned Google's success were funded by the public sector. The technology in the Apple iPhone was invented in the public sector. In both the US and Britain it was the state, not big pharma, that funded most ground-breaking 'new molecular entity' drugs, with the private sector then developing slight variations. And in Finland, it was the public sector that funded the early development of Nokia – and made a return on its investment."[29]

Since 1958, the US practice of allocating public resources to basic research for private gain has burgeoned, spurred initially by Soviet advances in rocket and satellite technology. The US Department of Energy has a $7-billion budget, 10 national laboratories, and thousands of government scientists to do basic physics research—research that will generate the technologies on which the innovations of the future will be based. The aim of this investment is to fill the new product funnel for US firms, including advanced weapons that will be sold to the Pentagon to bolster US military supremacy, so that the combined branches of the US armed services can continue to open foreign markets and keep them open. Washington spends vastly more on basic physics research than any other country—all to the benefit of US private enterprises and the investors who own them.

The US pharmaceutical industry is the beneficiary of Washington's—that is, US taxpayers'—$40 billion yearly investment in the National Institutes of Health. Every drug approved for sale by the US Food and Drug Administration from 2010 to 2016 was based on NIH-funded research.[30] Not only do drug companies benefit from government-funded research, they also receive generous tax breaks for the research they conduct in-house. This means taxpayers pay higher taxes in order to compensate for the taxes drug makers don't pay when they receive tax breaks for the research they conduct internally.

Another way capitalist governments intervene strongly in the economy to the benefit of investors is by creating markets. Markets, in the mythology of neoliberal economics, originate in the intersection of consumer needs and the energies of entrepreneurs to satisfy consumer needs in pursuit of private gain. It's all supposed to happen without government intervention. But often the state is both consumer and entrepreneur. Lockheed Martin, Raytheon, General Dynamics, Boeing, and Northrop Grumman, the United States' largest weapons-makers, wouldn't exist were it not for the billions of dollars the US government pays them every year for tools of war. These weapons are also purchased by US satellite countries, in the interests of ensuring their militaries achieve "interoperability" with US forces as part of US-led military alliances. Many of the advanced arms the Pentagon buys were developed by the Defense Advanced Research Projects Agency, based on publicly funded research. Public spending, then, is the keystone of the entire edifice. Taxpayers fund the development of new weapons systems and then buy them from private firms who manufacture them based on designs from publicly-funded labs. The arms dealers mark up the prices of the aircraft, warships, and tanks they make, to produce profits, which are then distributed as dividends to the firms' owners. The role of the owners is parasitic. Since arms manufacturing could be assigned to the public sector, as weapons R&D and procurement are, the only contribution the private owners make to the process is to collect a reward for their redundancy.

The US state also uses its power to distort arms markets to favor US providers. It does this by threatening to impose sanctions on countries that seek to buy weapons from US competitors. The Countering America's Adversaries Through Sanctions Act deters potential clients for Russian, Chinese, Iranian, and North Korean arms from dealing with the foreign rivals of Boeing, Raytheon, Lockheed Martin, and other US arms companies. For example, Washington threatened to sanction India if it bought missile defense systems from Russia, attempting to tilt the arms market toward US manufacturers. It has punished Turkey for buying a missile defense system from Russia. Coercing weapons buyers into purchasing from US arms dealers in preference to foreign ones, not only helps US arms manufacturers, but has the additional effect of reducing the economies of scale that rivals are able to achieve. This increases the expense of furnishing their own militaries with weapons, increasing their countries' defense burden.

Market creation by the state is not limited to weapons. The Canadian government has created a market for drug makers Moderna, Sanofi, and Resilience Biotechnologies, by guaranteeing orders for vaccine doses. Moderna will build an mRNA factory in Canada to produce 24 vaccines for different diseases, along with Covid-19 booster shots, and a shot that will combine Covid-19 and seasonal influenza vaccines. At the same time, Ottawa is giving Sanofi $415 million to build a vaccine manufacturing plant in Toronto, and $199 million to Resilience Biotechnologies to expand its facilities near Toronto. Resilience will produce 640 million mRNA vaccine doses yearly. Moderna, Sanofi, and Resilience would not produce vaccines in Canada without advance purchase agreements and injections of cash from Ottawa. Rather than investing in a state-owned pharmaceutical industry, the Canadian government—interconnected in manifold ways with its US patron in Washington and its own business community—prefers to shower foreign private enterprise with public Canadian funds.

Elon Musk's SpaceX and Jeff Bezos' Blue Origin have benefited from US government-created markets. Exploiting rocket technology developed in the public sector, they're raking in billions of dollars every year in government contracts. NASA will pay SpaceX approximately $9 billion to transport cargo and astronauts to the International Space Station, while the Pentagon pays the company $6 billion for rocket launches. Meanwhile, Blue Origin has won a contract to build a moon lander to return US astronauts to the moon as early as 2024.

Washington also engages in "market distorting" practices. For example, its "buy American" program constrains government procurement policy to favor US suppliers, even when foreign providers offer better quality or better pricing. This, in effect, acts as a subsidy to US firms. The Buy American Act requires that goods bought by the US government must contain at least 55 percent US content, rising to 75 percent by 2029.

The Biden administration has deceptively presented Buy American practices as recent departures from free market protocols—a "devil-made-me-do-it" response to a similar practice on China's part. But government procurement in favor of US firms has long antedated the United States' commercial rivalry with China. In 1920, the US Congress passed legislation, the Jones Act, still on the books, which requires ocean-going cargo transported to and from the continental USA to US colonies, such as Puerto Rico, to be carried by US-owned, crewed, registered and built vessels. The law creates a US monopoly over shipping, allowing US operators to exact monopoly fees from their clients. A shipping container transported from New York City to Puerto Rico—a protected route—costs over $3,000. The same shipment to Jamaica—an unprotected route, open to competition by non-US shippers—costs only half as much. The Jones Act is thus a subsidy to US shipping firms.[31]

Directives to buy from US companies are layered atop other legislation prohibiting US federal and state governments from buying specific goods from specific countries. For example, Congress passed a law in 2019 banning purchases by federal transportation authorities of railway cars and buses from Chinese-owned firms—to the advantage of non-Chinese manufacturers.

Washington also acts to ban foreign competitors from the US market, thereby protecting domestic providers. The cellphones and network equipment manufactured by the Chinese telecom manufacturer, Huawei, have been effectively banned from the US market on contrived national security grounds. Washington has shown itself to be perfectly willing to stretch national security considerations beyond credibility as a pretext to block foreign firms from access to the US market. The result is that US enterprise is sheltered from foreign competition.

Washington intervened in the "free market" in 2021 to protect the profit-making interests of US aerospace firms by pressuring Kiev to nationalize a Ukrainian aerospace manufacturer. While Washington professes opposition to nationalization, it enjoined the Ukrainian government to buy the firm to keep it out of the hands of a privately-owned Chinese aerospace enterprise. Washington was concerned that by buying the Ukrainian company, the Chinse business would absorb technology that would allow it to compete more effectively with its US rivals.

In a similar vein, the US state has intervened to distort the "free market" to prevent Chinese firms from winning contracts outside the United States. For example, the US International Development Finance Corp—a US agency that arranges credit for foreign governments and businesses to purchase goods and services from US providers, (yet another subsidy Washington provides Corporate USA)—has been offering "financial incentives and other enticements to countries willing to shun Chinese-made telecom gear."[32] The Development Finance Corp provided a $500-million loan to a consortium of telecom companies led by the UK's Vodaphone to build a mobile network in Ethiopia. A condition of the loan was that it would not be used to purchase Huawei equipment.[33] Meanwhile, Washington has given aid to Eastern European countries to build cellular networks, on the condition that only Huawei's rivals are used.[34] In effect, Washington is paying countries to spurn the Chinese supplier—a significant intrusion into the "free market."

The Development Finance Corp was created by Congress in 2018 to compete with China's One Belt, One Road initiative. While its main goal is to invest in US companies, the corporation is willing to support non-US firms, if doing so hurts Huawei. "We're not out to play defense," DFC head Adam Boehler told *The Wall Street Journal*. "We're out to play offense."[35] Offense means distorting markets, by using the power of the US state to eliminate Chinese firms, like Huawei. Washington's efforts in this regard, courtesy of the US taxpayer, have paid off. As *The Wall Street Journal* announced in a headline: "US Set Out to Hobble China's Huawei, and So It Has."[36]

On top of promoting Huawei's competitors, Washington has sought to degrade the company's products, by denying it access to US technology. In 2019, Washington banned the export of US-made chips to Huawei, and additionally blocked Huawei's access to chips made anywhere in the world with US equipment.

The aim, according to *The Wall Street Journal*'s editorial board, is to decouple "computer technology supply chains from China" and Huawei[37]—that is, to cripple Corporate USA's rivals.

Washington has also carried out a campaign of harassment against Huawei. According to the company, US officials instructed US "law enforcement to threaten, menace, coerce, entice and incite both current and former Huawei employees."[38] US prosecutors have brought charges of racketeering conspiracy and conspiring to steal trade secrets against Huawei and its partners. FBI agents have visited the homes of Huawei employees to pressure them to disclose information that could be used in US courts to hobble the telecom manufacturer.

In September 2021, the United States and European Union established a Trade and Technology Council to "seek to strengthen their competitiveness and technological leadership" while "developing common strategies to mitigate the impact of non-market practices," particularly in third-world countries, a reference widely interpreted to mean China. "Beijing's economic practices—including subsidies for favored industries—were one of the factors behind the commission's formation," reported *The Wall Street Journal*.[39] While calling out China for its use of subsidies, the United States and the European Union have long used subventions to bolster their own commercial airline industries. In the autumn of 2020, the World Trade Organization ruled "that both the US and EU provided prohibited subsidies to Boeing and Airbus, respectively."[40] The two governments imposed retaliatory tariffs on each other—yet another non-market action—but finally agreed to lift these measures in favor of building a common front against China, whose commercial airline manufacturing they see as a common threat to Boeing and Airbus. In his accustomed tendentious style, ruling class journalist "Scoop" Sanger wrote in *The New York Times* that the "United States had objected to government subsidies for private industry — whether it was Airbus in France or Huawei in China,"[41] failing to mention Washington's years-long subsidization of Boeing. He thereby reinforced the myth that the United States, seemingly alone

among large powers, favors a free-market, while its economic competitors are continually cheating by subsidizing their enterprises.

While the Trade and Technology Council condemned what
it called "distortive industrial subsidies" and vowed to coordinate action against them, it was clear that the only subsidies the
United States and the European Union objected to were those
of third-world countries, and China's in particular. On top of all
the usual subsidies the United States had already lavished upon
Corporate USA, the Biden administration was, at the same time
it was coordinating with the European Union to retaliate against
China's subsidies, rolling out "the most expansive industrial policy
legislation in US history," proposing to make a "nearly quarter-tril-
lion-dollar investment in building up America's manufacturing and
technological edge,"[42] by means of a panoply of new subsidies. Biden
was engineering the greatest subsidy program in human history, all
the while denouncing Beijing's program of subventions.

As *The Wall Street Journal* explained, Washington was "pre-
paring to direct government power and policy toward building up
domestic capacity in" semiconductors, critical minerals, medical
supplies and battery technologies via direct government investment, tax incentives for private investment, and removal of regulatory barriers.[43] Biden also proposed to spend $400 billion on
infrastructure projects that would use US products; to allocate $300
billion to research and development of new products—filling the
new product funnel for private enterprise; and to enhance the Berry
Amendment which directs the military to buy from US firms.[44] Of
these, the second was perhaps the most noteworthy. Washington
was proposing to take on the burden—more precisely, it was planning to have taxpayers take on the burden—of developing new
products for private firms and the enrichment of the firms' owners,
members of the same class to which the Biden administration is
intimately connected.

With regard to semiconductors, US legislators proposed to
fund research into their design and production; subsidize the
construction of semiconductor manufacturing facilities in the

United States; and provide tax credits to US-based semiconductor manufacturers.[45] On top of these subsidies and favors for US business, Washington would also spend "$100 billion over five years for research into artificial intelligence and machine learning, robotics, high-performance computing and other advanced technologies,"[46] according to *The Wall Street Journal*, the fruits of which would be used by Corporate USA for its own aggrandizement.

The Biden administration even proposed a new agency along the Defense Advanced Research Projects Agency's lines to produce basic science in healthcare, the Advanced Research Projects Agency for Health. Working under the aegis of the National Institutes of Health, the agency would undertake basic research on Alzheimer's, cancer, diabetes, and potential pandemic pathogens. It would receive funding of $6.5 billion per year.[47]

Harvard health economist Amitabh Chandra explained that taxpayers needed to fund basic research to produce life-saving and disease-preventing innovations because the private sector won't do it. "A lot of basic science is not profitable. It's just knowledge. At some point basic science becomes useful, and then the private sector can come in."[48] In other words, new drugs and therapies aren't produced by pharmaceutical entrepreneurs who risk their capital in the pursuit of the complementary goals of serving humanity and growing rich. The truth of the matter is that the public sector does the heavy lifting and when it has produced a potentially profitable innovation, the private sector swoops in—with full government approval—to reap the rewards. Chandra didn't raise the obvious question: Why not eliminate the private sector and let the public sector handle the process from basic research to distribution?

Enlisting public funds to produce innovations that can be transferred to the private sector is not limited to medical research: it is the foundation of a vast nanny state for private enterprises—one that spans multiple industries, from pharmaceuticals to computing, aircraft to electric vehicles. As Senate Majority leader Chuck Schumer explained, Washington invests taxpayer funds in the products and industries of tomorrow, and then lets "the private sector take that knowledge and create jobs."[49] What he really meant is create profits. The public sector could just as easily create jobs out of the knowledge it has, itself, produced, without transferring the knowledge to the billionaire class. This would have the advantage of unburdening the public of the oppressive weight of billionaires it bears upon its shoulders.

***

The United States is a model of state-directed economics as much as is China. It simply pretends otherwise. It bids other countries, and at times coerces them at the point of a gun or under the threat of starvation, to do as it says it does rather than as it actually does. So it is that George W. Bush could sing paeans to free-trade, while in the same breath announce steel tariffs. Barack Obama could rhapsodize about how the US "free-enterprise system drives innovation," and then add that "throughout history our government has provided cutting-edge scientists and inventors with the support that they need" because it is not "profitable for companies to invest in basic research."[50]

The difference between US- and Chinese-state-directed economics is that a micro-elite of wealthy US shareholders, investors, and bankers, acting through a power elite in government, uses the US state to steer the US economy in directions that protect and promote their interests, while in China, the Communist party steers the Chinese economy in directions that protect and promote the economic development interests of the Chinese people as a whole. In the former case, state-directed economics is yoked to the interests of a US financial class as a project of minority wealth expansion; in the latter, it is yoked to the project of China's national rejuvenation. While the models are alike, the differences in the aims are illustrated in this observation from *The Wall Street Journal*: "A figure like [Apple Inc. Tim] Cook commands a great deal of respect, even deference, in Washington. In Beijing, he's treated like any other business executive—as a supplicant, angling for favors to keep his market hopes alive."[51] In the United States, capitalism is an end in itself. In China, it's the means to an end.

The implication for public health emergencies is that if capitalism is in command the response will reflect capitalist interests. If profits aren't in command, governments have the latitude to act in the public interest.

CHAPTER 5

CAPITALIST PHARMACY

*Instead of society undertaking to reckon up what it needs
and how much of each article, the factory owners
simply produce upon the calculation of what will bring them
the most profit.* — N. Bukharin and E. Preobrazhensky[1]

On an autumn day in 2021, Merck, the giant US pharmaceutical company, announced a breakthrough. It was ready to seek approval for an antiviral pill to be used in the treatment of Covid-19. The new drug, according to the preliminary results of a phase 3 clinical trial, reduced the chances of hospitalization by 50 percent among patients with mild to moderate disease. Monoclonal antibody treatment, developed by Regeneron and GlaxoSmithKline, was already available for non-hospitalized patients, but required patients to travel to a hospital for an infusion and was therefore considered too time consuming and resource-intensive to be practical. Popping a pill would be much easier.

Merck's announcement was greeted with considerable enthusiasm in the business press. A new drug in the armamentarium of compounds to treat Covid-19 would help protect hospitals and medical resources from undue strain as countries moved away from elimination and mitigation to uncontrolled transmission and a return to business normal.

Additionally, the new drug meshed perfectly with the capitalist zeitgeist. Apart from promising a cornucopia of profits for Merck and its shareholders, it helped solve the problem of how to open the economy to profit-making amid a pandemic, without crashing healthcare systems. Plus, it resonated with the preference of capitalist medicine for treatment over prevention.

For investors, disease is an opportunity—a problem crying out for a solution. Those who offer solutions have a chance to turn their capital into more capital. Prevention, however, is not opportunity. It is, on the contrary, opportunity's nemesis. No drug maker ever got rich in a country of robustly healthy people. The sad reality for drug companies and health insurers is that people who stay healthy through regular exercise, a salubrious diet, and the blessings of a generously funded public health body, present few profit-making opportunities. To prosper, pharmaceutical companies need disease—real, imagined, or contrived.

The world's failure to prevent a pandemic by acting quickly and decisively to impose public health measures became an opportunity for drug companies. That's not to say that pharmaceutical companies actively discouraged prevention, but prevention is often discouraged all the same if the availability of therapeutics makes prevention an option rather than necessity. For example, diet modification and other lifestyle changes may be the best way to deal with gastritis. But the existence of proton pump inhibitors—drugs used to reduce stomach acid—makes it easy for gastritis-sufferers to avoid the inconvenient tasks of modifying their diets and changing their lifestyles. Likewise, the promise of vaccines and therapies made it easier to avoid the costs of implementing non-pharmaceutical public health measures. Instead, it could be said—as Anthony Fauci did say— that the cavalry (meaning vaccines and therapeutics) was coming. Waiting for a pharmaceutical cavalry to arrive also had the congenial outcome for capitalists of creating an Eldorado of profit-making opportunities in pharmaceutical and biotechnology concerns.

The cost to produce Merck's antiviral pill, which the company named Molnupiravir, was $17.74 per treatment, according to the online investigative journalism site, *The Intercept*.[2] One treatment—which would consist of eight pills taken daily over five days, or 40 pills in total—would cost $712, over 40 times the cost of production.

It wasn't long before Merck's profiteering was attacked. Critics pointed out that the treatment's exorbitant price would put the drug out of reach for most people who needed it. Moreover, few people would be inclined to pay over $700 for a course of treatment to relieve symptoms that were only mild to moderate. This was definitely a drug for the wealthy, priced to maximize Merck's profits, not to help humanity.

The drug had been developed by George Painter, a professor in the department of pharmacology and chemical biology at Emory University, with a grant from the US Department of Defense. Painter developed the drug for soldiers to take if they were exposed to weaponized equine encephalitis, a pathogen developed by US and Soviet researchers as a bioweapon. Recognizing the drug's possible application to Covid-19, the compound's license was acquired by Ridgeback Pharmaceuticals, which partnered with Merck to take advantage of the latter's manufacturing scale. Hence, neither Merck nor Ridgeback had anything to do with the drug's development. It was entirely the invention of an anonymous university researcher funded by the US government.[3] Anthony Fauci's National Institute of Allergy and Infectious Diseases also chipped in. Plus, Merck received a generous $1.2 billion pre-order of the drug from Washington before the treatment had even been approved by regulators. Sales were expected to reach $7 billion by the end of 2021 alone.

Dzintars Gotham, a physician at King's College Hospital in the United Kingdom, remarked that: "It's a great coup that the American government funded some scientists to develop antivirals. The great tragedy is that, after their great success, they just gave it away to private industry with apparently no strings attached."[4]

Gotham may not have known that the great tragedy was hardly an anomaly. Transferring publicly-created pharmaceutical knowledge to private industry is the way things normally get done in the world of capitalist pharmacy. Indeed, the development and pricing of Molnupiravir was emblematic of how capitalist pharmacy works. The state takes dollars out of taxpayers' pockets and puts scientists into university and government labs to produce drugs for private pharmaceutical firms, which price the treatments based not on what's good for the health of the taxpayers who funded them, but on what's good for the health of the portfolios of their investors.

When capitalism's pleasing clothing is stripped away and its nakedness exposed, there are few people who are not revolted by its ugliness, no less so in the manufacture of drugs. Those not revolted are the people who benefit most handsomely from this affront against humanity. Thefts from the public purse; price gouging and profiteering; indifference to the health of others in the amoral pursuit of profit; these are aspects of capitalist pharmacy. They call forth the greatest indignation, revealing a truth. However much the public believes it is pro-capitalist, it is, despite its suspicion of the word "socialism," committed to the values socialism embodies. Were this not true, most people wouldn't recoil from the idea that it is acceptable for drug companies to base their pricing upon the calculation of what will bring them the greatest profit.

**

Capitalist pharmacy exists for one reason alone—to generate profits. It drives inexorably toward the protection and promotion of the financial health of its investors, not the physical and mental health of its customers. Once this key reality is understood, capitalist pharmacy is understood.

In a rationally planned economy, we would want the pharmaceutical industry to produce the drugs people need in quantities sufficient to meet significant health needs. We would also want it to develop new drugs to satisfy significant unmet health needs. Additionally, we would want it to distribute treatments according to need, so that all who could benefit, do benefit. In other words, society would undertake to reckon up what it needs and how much of each drug, and then produce what is needed within the constraints of available resources. But in a society organized around the production of profit, this doesn't happen. Instead, the industry's owners simply produce upon the calculation of what will bring them the greatest material gain.

The yoking of the pharmaceutical industry to the capitalist imperative of producing a profit forces the industry to depart from the path of rational planning aimed at maximizing public value in favor of maximizing shareholder value. As a consequence, capitalist pharmacy accepts the following limitations as the *sine qua non* of achieving its profit-making mission.

- It focuses only on the most profitable drugs, even when they contribute little or nothing to public health, or in fact harm it, while at the same time avoiding investment in drugs that would satisfy significant unmet health needs, but which have low or uncertain financial payoffs.
- It focuses only on the most profitable markets, ignoring demographic segments and countries where consumers have limited incomes and are unlikely to be able to afford prices which support large profit-margins.
- It commits to delivering shareholder value now, shunning long term investments in the development of drugs in favor of quick hits with immediate payoffs. If important therapies require long term investment, they are avoided, and assigned to the public sector.

The perfect drug from the point of view of the capitalist pharmaceutical industry is a compound that costs little to produce, or whose development has been subsidized by the public, and which patients take daily for a lifetime to manage a disease of affluence but not to cure it. Drugs that match this profile are the industry's "blockbusters," and include compounds for such chronic conditions as diabetes and high cholesterol and especially life-long treatments, like thyroid medication, that produce ongoing revenue streams.

"Pharmaceutical companies tend to give priority to drugs that are taken daily, not once or twice in a lifetime,"[5] observes infectious disease expert Paul A. Offit. And they certainly don't give priority to drugs that cure or prevent disease. These drugs, in the words of an industry analyst, are a bad business model.[6] A drug that cures a disease destroys future demand. So too do drugs, like vaccines, which prevent disease. The pharmaceutical industry exists to create profits by offering solutions to real, imagined, or invented problems. Solutions that eliminate problems altogether, eliminate the reason for the industry to exist. Capitalists don't deliberately commit suicide. They seek to produce products and services that manage problems without preventing or eliminating them.

Until the coronavirus came along, vaccines were increasingly shunned by pharmaceutical companies as unprofitable. On the eve of the Covid-19 pandemic, only four large drug makers were still in the business of making vaccines: Merck, Sanofi, Pfizer, and Johnson & Johnson. Vaccines are an unattractive business model because they are often unaffordable to those who can benefit from them, and because they rarely generate ongoing revenue streams. Vaccines are normally intended either for: (1) diseases that afflict the extremely poor (schistosomiasis, Chagas disease, leishmaniasis), who lack the income to pay for the vaccines; (2) for stockpiling against pandemic threats (in which case, the demand is limited to whatever is necessary to fill the stockpile); (3) for epidemics that may gutter out before the vaccine is produced. (For example, by the time a vaccine against SARS had been developed, the SARS outbreak had ended). Additionally, vaccines are intended for outbreaks that the vaccines may very well end, denying the vaccine maker future revenue streams. Vaccines that eliminate disease are the equivalent of a washing machine that never breaks down.

On top of this, vaccines are expensive and time-consuming to develop. There is a high risk of failure at every stage of development. Additionally, the compounds carry heavy legal risks related to the possibility that recipients will be injured or killed by adverse side-effects. And because they are seen as a public good, pharmaceutical companies are pressured to provide vaccines at a low cost. For these reasons, vaccines are viewed by the pharmaceutical industry as poor profit-making opportunities. Indeed, as Bill Gates explained, without significant intervention by the public sector, the capitalist pharmaceutical industry would never have manufactured Covid-19 vaccines. "You can't call up Johnson & Johnson or AstraZeneca and say, 'Hey, here's a chance to lose $500 million.'"[7] Because vaccines are normally money-losing ventures, governments had to step in to organize the production of Covid-19 shots. Yoked to the pursuit of private gain, capitalist pharmacy was not up to the task. This explains why a universal flu vaccine—a single shot to confer lifetime immunity against influenza—remains an unrealized potential.

***

The influenza virus resembles a head of broccoli. Owing to ongoing mutations, the morphology of the head changes from season to season. Since seasonal vaccines target the head, they must be reformulated every year to home in on the shape-shifting virus. This works out well for flu vaccine manufacturers. Mutation guarantees an ongoing revenue stream. But the influenza virus, like a broccoli head, also has a stalk. Unlike the head, the stalk changes slowly. A vaccine that targeted the stalk rather than the protean head would only need to be taken once—or at most a few times in a lifetime. This would obviate the need to schedule a flu shot every year. And it would save the collective expense of disbursing funds from the public purse annually to vaccine makers—funds that could be more efficiently used for other purposes. Of course, a universal flu vaccine would harm a very tiny fraction of the public, namely investors with financial stakes in the pharmaceutical companies that produce seasonal flu vaccines.

A universal flu vaccine has been a possibility for decades. Nevertheless, one has yet to be developed. John Barry, an historian who wrote a best-selling book about the Great Influenza of 1918-

1920, notes that developing a universal influenza vaccine ought to be one of humanity's highest priorities because the avian flu is among humanity's greatest threats. All the same, few resources have been allocated to the project.[8] Florian Krammer, a virologist at the Icahn School of Medicine in New York City, notes that "If you had Operation Warp Speed for universal flu vaccines you might already have one."[9] The author, journalist, and academic Mike Davis concurs. According to Davis, "Virtually all researchers agree that the tools exist to fashion a broadband vaccine that incapacitates the invariant stalks, thus conferring general immunity against all strains that might last for years. The research is out there, but Big Pharma won't develop or manufacture such a vaccine because it is not profitable." Davis argues that a universal vaccine would violate the capitalist imperative of creating planned obsolescence. "If given a radical design for a car that lasts for a lifetime," he asks, "would GM manufacture it?"[10] By the same token, bringing to fruition the promise inherent in science's ability to produce a universal influenza vaccine would threaten pharmaceutical industry profits. Drug companies would rather pump out new flu vaccines every year to guarantee revenue streams far into the future than develop a universal flu shot that would only have to be taken once, even if sacrificing future revenue streams means protecting humanity from one of its most significant viral threats. A global avian flu outbreak would likely wipe out some 300 million human beings,[11] making the Covid-19 pandemic look like a walk in the park. It is within our capability to inoculate everyone against a potential influenza horror. Capitalism, however, presents this possibility as a threat to the profit-making interests of Big Pharma, and so humanity as a whole is sacrificed to a miniscule fraction of its number.

***

Antibiotics are another class of drugs whose development fails to accord with the incentive structure of capitalist pharmacy.

An antibiotic's useful life is limited by the reality that bacteria evolve, and eventually become resistant. This means that antibiotics have to be continually reinvented, a process that involves incurring new development costs. Since the average drug costs $1.4 billion to develop, and only 14 percent of antibiotics ever pan out in clinical trials, antibiotics are not congenial to pharmaceutical industry profit-making.

Relatively few people have infections that are resistant to existing antibiotics, and therefore the market for new antibiotics is small. As we've seen, drug companies prefer to develop formulations that can treat conditions that many people have, even if the ailments are mild, non-life threatening, and more of an inconvenience than a threat.

In order to slow the development of antibiotic resistance, physicians have developed a protocol, called antibiotic stewardship, to use these drugs sparingly. This, of course, limits sales and makes the drugs unattractive to pharmaceutical companies. John Rex, a physician and drug developer, sums up the problem this way: No one will use a bad antibiotic. But in order to conserve a good one, physicians will rarely use it.[12]

Because the incentive structure of capitalist pharmacy militates against private industry developing antibiotics, the US government has used its guiding hand to contrive non-market incentives to induce private firms to act in a manner that conduces to the public weal. Because capitalism can't do it, the government must. To keep the antibiotic industry alive, the US government uses a duo of push and pull incentives. Push incentives are public funding for research and development. Pull incentives are advance purchase agreements.

The US government's Biomedical Advanced Research and Development Authority, or BARDA, provides push grants to private firms to stimulate research on antibiotics. It has provided a pull incentive to the drug company, Paratek, in the form of a $285-million advance purchase agreement for doses of omadacycline, an antibiotic used by the military to protect troops from weaponized anthrax.

These, as we'll see, are the same government-created incentives the Trump administration used to induce capitalist pharmaceutical companies to develop Covid-19 vaccines. They are also the same incentives that were used to incent Merck to produce the antiviral pill, Molnupiravir.

**

If capitalist pharmacy is partial to drugs that are taken daily to manage chronic conditions rather than to cure or prevent them, it is also partial to consumers with lots of money who are in a position to pay high prices for the pharmaceutical companies' wares. Conversely, capitalist pharmaceutical companies steer clear of poverty, even though it is often within poverty that the most significant unmet health needs are found.

In the first decade of the twenty-first century, only 4 percent of newly approved drugs targeted diseases that mainly afflicted low- and middle-income countries.[13] Because capitalism is a barrier to the development of drugs to relieve conditions that afflict poor countries, development of these drugs depends on charitable donations to non-profit NGOs, such as the Drugs for Neglected Diseases *initiative* (DND*i*), known sardonically as Drugs for Diseases Neglected by Capitalist Medicine. The paucity of investment in malaria compared with diseases that are more common in rich countries has been one of the reasons why a malaria vaccine has been so long in the making. It has taken 30 years to produce an anti-malarial vaccine for children.[14] Because rich consumers have the means to pay high drug prices and poor people don't, capitalist pharmacy favors drugs such as cholesterol-lowering statins for overfed rich people, while eschewing the development of treatments for underfed poor people.

The drive for profit also constrains capitalist pharmacy in another way: Executives are under incessant pressure to pare back research and development to maximize allocation of net revenue to buying back shares, and investing in marketing. Share buybacks

produce immediate gains: they drive up a firm's share price, bene-
fitting shareholders, as well as the company's executive officers,
who are often compensated in shares. In contrast, the same dollar
invested in research and development may never payoff—and
if it does, it will likely do so years down the road. According to
the Pharmaceutical Research and Manufacturers of America, on
average, a new drug takes 10 to 15 years to develop and costs $2.6
billion. Most new drugs never make it to market.[15] Clearly, there
are strong incentives to shift net revenue to share buybacks and
away from R&D.

R&D also competes with marketing. Spending a dollar to adver-
tise a drug to treat erectile dysfunction—a condition that can often
be treated non-pharmaceutically—will likely produce a greater
payoff in a shorter time than spending the same dollar researching
a drug to satisfy a significant unmet health need. Clearly, incentives
to shift net revenue to marketing and away from R&D are just as
strong as they are to spend lavishly on driving up share prices.

Regarding marketing, if drug manufacturers are making drugs
to make sick people well, why do the drugs need to be advertised
and promoted? Surely, little effort is required to persuade consumers with significant unmet health needs of the benefit of drugs that
treat their condition safely and effectively. And yet drug companies
spend hundreds of millions of dollars on marketing. The reason why
is because a lot of the drugs that pharmaceutical companies make
are either not needed, or treat conditions that consumers don't care
about. Consumers must, therefore, be convinced they need them.

From 2009-2018, the 18 pharmaceutical companies listed on
the S&P 500 spent more on share buybacks ($335 billion) and divi-
dends ($287 billion) together than they did on R&D ($544 billion).[16]
Over the past decade, the giant US pharmaceutical company, Pfizer,
spent more on share buybacks and dividends ($139 billion) than
R&D ($82 billion.) [17]

***

In June, 2021, the US Food and Drug Administration—the body that regulates the sale of drugs in the United States—approved a drug for the treatment of Alzheimer's disease. Developed by Biogen, the drug is called Aducanumab. Analysts predicted the compound would become a blockbuster—a highly priced drug that would not cure, but would be used to manage, a chronic condition, producing a rich stream of revenue for Biogen stretching far into the future. At a cost of $56,000 per year, the drug was indeed pricey. That was one reason it promised to be a goldmine for the company and its shareholders—or so analysts expected.

There was only one problem: Aducanumab didn't work.

Biogen had conducted two trials, both of which were stopped when an independent data monitoring committee concluded the drug had no effect in reducing Alzheimer's symptoms. One trial showed the drug produced no discernible improvement in patients. A second produced data that showed at high doses the drug produced a very small reduction in cognitive decline—less than half a point on an 18-point scale. But this miniscule improvement was achieved at the expense of creating harm. Some 40 percent of participants in the trial who received a high dose experienced brain swelling or bleeding.

In November 2020, the FDA's independent advisory committee strongly recommended against approval. When the agency approved the drug anyway, three members of the committee resigned in protest.

The FDA's biostatistical office concluded "there is no compelling, substantial evidence of treatment effect or disease slowing."[18] The American Neurological Association recommended against approval. A former Biogen senior medical director, Dr. Vissia Viglietta, who was involved in designing the clinical trials, said: "This approval shouldn't have happened. It defeats everything I believe in scientifically and it lowers the rigor of regulatory bodies."[19] Dr. G. Caleb Alexander, a drug safety and effectiveness expert who was on the FDA advisory committee intoned, "This product, even in the best of circumstances, would be not terribly effective at all, with significant safety risks."[20] Even the regulator acknowledged there was no evidence the drug works.

So why did the drug garner FDA approval? The regulatory body said it approved Aducanumab because there is an Alzheimer's treatment vacuum that needs to be filled. In other words, in the regulator's view, an ineffective and harmful drug is preferable to no drug at all. But who would prefer a harmful drug that doesn't work to no drug? The obvious answer—Biogen's shareholders. It is difficult to avoid the conclusion that the FDA acted in the interests of private interests at the public's expense.

For years, scientists had entertained the hypothesis that Alzheimer's is caused by an accumulation of a substance called beta-amyloid. A drug that eliminates build-ups of the substance might slow cognitive decline. But a number of drugs developed to do just that, failed. Pfizer gave up its search for an Alzheimer's drug, laying off 300 employees. But Biogen, attracted by the allure of a potential Eldorado, persisted. When the company's early stage studies showed promising results, investors flocked to the company, driving up its share price. And when late stage trials failed to pan out, analysts said it was the knell of the beta amyloid hypothesis, adding that it was never well thought out anyway. And then the FDA intervened, to resurrect Biogen's dreams of pharaonic wealth.

Slowing cognitive decline in Alzheimer's patients is a significant unmet health need. Resources ought to be allocated to satisfying this need. But the FDA approved Biogen's Alzheimer's drug to satisfy, not an unmet health need, but Biogen's unmet need for a blockbuster drug that would serve as a goldmine for its shareholders.

In the end, Biogen may be denied its blockbuster drug. Aware that clinical trials have shown the drug to be marginally effective at best, and more likely harmful and completely useless, insurance companies, driven by their own profit-imperative, refused to cover the drug. The expert panel advising the European Union's drug regulator, recommended against approving the drug for sale in Europe. The Alzheimer's Society of Canada said that approving the drug for use in Canada could not be justified. In December 2021, 18 scientists signed a statement demanding the FDA rescind its decision to approve Aducanumab. In response, Biogen slashed the annual price of its drug in half, from $56,000 to $28,000.[21]

"Biogen has said it expects Medicare, the health insurance program for elderly and disabled people, to cover over 80 percent of the roughly one million to two million US Alzheimer's patients who could benefit from the drug."[22] If true, Biogen would plunder the public purse, robbing taxpayers of funds that could be used to underwrite coverage of treatments that actually make a difference, while placing patients at risk of brain bleeds and hemorrhages.

The moral of the Aducanumab story is that capitalist pharmacy is driven to make products that generate profit, not drugs that are safe and effective. Under a system in which profit is alpha and omega, safety and efficacy are preferable, but not essential. The second moral is that regulators—many of whom have strong ties to the industry—cannot be counted on to protect the public interest against the profit-making imperatives of capitalist pharmacy.

***

Merck's Molnupiravir, the antiviral pill touted as a breakthrough with the capability to reduce the number of patients that need to be hospitalized with Covid-19, turned out to be very much like Aducanumab. Its efficacy was unimpressive, there was reason to believe it was dangerous, and yet, despite the reservations about the drug expressed by a number of scientists, regulators were prepared to give the pills their imprimatur.

Molnupiravir works by scrambling a virus's genetic code, interfering with its ability to replicate. A number of scientists worried that the drug might also induce genetic changes in patients' own cells, causing cancers, genetic diseases, and birth defects. Merck's own research suggested the potential for mutations.[23] Scientists also feared that Molnupiravir could engender genetic modifications in the novel coronavirus that would make the pathogen more transmissible or deadly. Indeed, FDA scientists found troubling mutations in viral samples taken from trial participants.[24]

What's more, while preliminary trial results suggested the drug could cut hospitalization rates by 50 percent, the completed study showed that hospitalization rates were reduced by only 30 percent. In fact, the second half of the study showed that those who took the drug were no less likely to stay out of the hospital than trial participants who received a placebo.[25] According to Sally Hunsberger, a statistician at the Biometrics Research Branch of the National Institute of Allergy and Infectious Diseases, the benefits were "pretty minimal."[26]

Why, then, would regulators approve a drug that might cause cancer and other illnesses, might produce new variants against which the current crop of Covid-19 vaccines is powerless, and which, for most people, has no effect in preventing hospitalization? Moreover, why would Washington agree to pay Merck over $700 per treatment for a drug that costs only $17 to make,[27] especially given concerns about its safety and efficacy?

As in the case of Aducanumab, so too with Molnupiravir: capitalist pharmacy is driven to produce products that generate profit, not drugs that are safe and effective. Capitalist governments facilitate the drug companies' profit-making, not only by approving drugs of dubious safety and efficacy, but by buying them at grossly inflated prices.

***

Patents are often the principal target for critics of capitalist pharmacy. Drug patents are temporary monopolies, typically lasting 20 years. Patent holders have exclusive commercial rights to a drug, method, or technology. They can license their invention to another party, typically for a fee.

The principal benefit of a patent is that it allows holders to set whatever price they want, paving the way to Pantagruelian profits. Drugs protected by a patent tend to be set very high—15 times higher on average than compounds that are patent-free.[28] Gilead's Sofosbuvir-based therapy for hepatitis C costs $84,000 per treatment. CordenPharma's Lomustine, an anti-cancer drug, is sold at an exorbitant $768 per pill. Otsuka Pharmaceutical's Deltyba, an anti-tuberculosis drug, costs $1,700 per treatment. Pfizer's phenytoin sodium, an anti-epilepsy drug, costs $90 per 100 mg pack.

Exorbitant monopoly prices are said to be necessary to encourage innovation by allowing patent holders to recover their research and development costs. But this assumes that R&D costs are substantial. They may not be. Often R&D costs are borne by the public. Typically, the cost of developing new drugs is shared between governments and private enterprise. Basic research is done in government labs or publicly-funded universities. Clinical trials—the experiments to test new drugs for safety and efficacy—are paid for by the pharmaceutical companies. Governments pay as much as two-thirds of all R&D costs.[29] In the United States, the National Institutes of Health invest over $40 billion annually in medical research. Of new drugs approved by the Food and Drug Administration from 2010 to 2016, all were based on research conducted in the public sector.

In a rationally planned economy, the price of pharmaceuticals would be set to recover costs. But patents go beyond cost recovery. By creating a monopoly, the patent holder is able to price to maximize profits, even if that means pricing beyond the means of many people who could benefit from the drug. Drug companies, then, don't set prices to recover their cost and return a modest profit. They set prices to recover their cost and return as high a profit as they possibly can, even if most of the people who could benefit from the treatment are priced out of the market.

Patent laws incent drug companies to focus their efforts on drugs that are potentially patentable, since these drugs can be sheltered from competition and priced to produce monopoly profits. At the same time, they discourage pharmaceutical companies from carrying out research on drugs whose patents have expired. Some drugs may be effective in treating conditions other than those for which they were originally patented. Drug companies, however, are uninterested in exploring potential applications of drugs to other conditions, if the drugs' patents are no longer valid.

Patent laws also encourage "evergreening," the practice of introducing minor modifications to a drug, and then declaring it a new invention, so that it can be re-patented. This encourages drug companies to focus their research on minor modifications to existing drugs with a high level of demand. The corollary is that drug makers don't invest in developing new therapies to satisfy unmet medical needs. Instead, they leave this vital job to the public sector.

The policy of the US government is to license federally owned patents—that is, inventions created in government labs—to private enterprise for commercial exploitation, a practice called "technology transfer." This is an obvious boon for drug companies, since it allows them to capitalize on the basic science carried out by the public sector. Messenger RNA technology developed in US government laboratories was foundational to Moderna and BioNTech, Pfizer's partner, to produce their Covid-19 vaccines. The technology is pregnant with the promise of applications well beyond the novel coronavirus, including cancer treatment, regeneration of heart tissue in patients with heart failure, repair of tissue damage due to aging, and vaccines for influenza, Zika, HIV, Epstein-Barr, CMV, and other diseases. The transfer of this technology from the public sector to private enterprise betokens years of Himalayan riches for the billionaire class, courtesy of taxpayers.

***

Patents came under attack in 2020 when it became clear that, with only a few companies manufacturing Covid-19 vaccines, it would take years to produce enough vaccines to inoculate everyone in the world. While rich countries vaccinated their adult populations quickly, and even began to offer booster shots, despite the absence of evidence that boosters were needed to prevent severe illness and hospitalization, people in low- and middle-income countries were left at the back of the queue. It was estimated that poor countries would not be fully vaccinated until 2024.

The World Health Organization beseeched the United States and the European Union to suspend their plans to offer booster shots, and instead to send their surplus doses to the global south, where even most healthcare workers and other members of high-risk populations had not been vaccinated.

There were two compelling reasons to accelerate vaccine distribution: First, to overcome the moral failure of a vaccine apartheid, where the world's rich were protected and its poor neglected. Second, to get everyone in the world vaccinated as quickly as possible to prevent the emergence of new viral variants that might elude the protection offered by the existing set of vaccines.

To get more shots into more arms, more vaccine doses would be needed. But that was a problem since Pfizer, BioNTech, Moderna, AstraZeneca, and Johnson & Johnson, the vaccine producers in the West, were adamantly opposed to waiving their patents and sharing their vaccine know-how with other manufacturers. And so too were most Western governments.

Some governments, public health officials, and advocates argued that if patent rights were temporarily suspended and other manufacturers were allowed to produce generic copies of the vaccines, the vaccine supply would greatly expand, significantly hastening the roll-out of inoculations to the world, accelerating the end of the pandemic, and saving millions of lives.

But the vaccine makers—and the governments with which they were interlocked—were adamant in their opposition. The reasons why were fairly obvious. First, the waiving of patent rights and transfer of technology would significantly reduce the drug companies' revenue from vaccine sales. They had no motivation to divide the world market with other manufacturers—even if it meant the world would be fully vaccinated sooner, with significant benefits for all. Second, Pfizer and Moderna viewed their mRNA technology as the basis for applications beyond Covid-19 and a future cornucopia of profits. Moderna had multiple mRNA vaccines under development, aimed at other respiratory viruses, tropical viruses, and HIV. Neither Moderna nor Pfizer were prepared to disclose their trade secrets to competitors, since these were the basis of their future prosperity. As regards the dangers of "vaccine escape"—the emergence of new viral variants against which the current array of vaccines would be powerless—this was, for the profit-driven vaccine makers, less a concern than an opportunity. Vaccine escape would produce a never-ending stream of revenue, as new vaccine formulations would be needed to combat the mutating virus.

A majority of countries backed an emergency resolution at the World Trade Organization, sponsored by India and South Africa, to waive patents on Covid-19 vaccines. While Washington initially opposed the resolution, it later reversed its position. Washington's *volte-face* was a public relations gambit intended to burnish its reputation, and not a meaningful expression of support for the resolution. The WTO operates by consensus. Everyone must agree, and European countries, especially Germany, along with other governments in the world, including Canada's, were vehemently opposed. Washington could safely say it was for the resolution, knowing the proposal would never be ratified.

Even if it was approved, manufacturers would require more than waived patents to produce generic copies of the Pfizer-BioNTech, Moderna, AstraZeneca, and Johnson & Johnson vaccines. They would also require the know-how, to say nothing of special equipment. The vaccine makers could refuse to share these essentials. Indeed, Moderna categorically declined to share its recipe, offering instead to significantly ramp up its production to provide free doses to poor countries. However, as of mid-October 2021, the company hadn't followed through on its promise, diverting additional doses instead to high-income countries that were willing to pay top dollars for booster shots, or to poor countries willing to pay for doses rather than waiting for donations.[30]

Finally, the US government held the patent that Pfizer had licensed through its partner BioNTech, and it also claimed a patent on the Moderna vaccine as co-inventor. If it so desired, it could have licensed the patents to generic vaccine makers. It chose not to.

What's more, the White House could have used its powers under the Defense Production Act, a 1950 law that gives the president broad powers over US companies in emergency situations, to force vaccine makers to share their intellectual property with other manufacturers. It didn't do this. Washington, then, despite withdrawing its opposition to patent waivers on Covid-19 vaccines, had no genuine interest in accelerating vaccine production by encouraging the manufacture of generics. It was practising duplicity.

***

Patents are lightning rods for Big Pharma's sharpest critics, but even if patents were waived on all drugs permanently, capitalist pharmacy would still be capitalist and therefore burdened by capitalism's ills. Drug companies would continue to parasitize the public sector as the source of their new products. Drug prices would be lower, but drugs would still be treated as commodities—that is, as items produced to turn a profit, not to satisfy the public's need for medications to safeguard and improve health. Supply shortages, such as the Covid-19 vaccine shortage which impeded the rapid vaccination of all humanity, would be less likely to occur. But drug prices would still include a profit component, necessary to satisfy share- and bond-holders, whose contribution as providers of capital to the development and manufacture of drugs could be readily replaced by the public sector, and whose parasitism as collectors of dividends and interest is harmful and larcenous.

In a rationally planned society, in which drugs are produced to satisfy important health needs, costs would be recovered out of the public purse, within the constraints of the efficient allocation of limited resources among multiple competing demands. This contrasts with the capitalist practice of recovering costs plus an additional amount for profits by pricing as high as possible, even if doing so means a substantial proportion of those who need the drug are unable to pay. It also contrasts with the capitalist practice of producing drugs that are useless and even harmful, or are intended to relieve conditions that can be more effectively or efficiently treated in less expensive ways, so long as they produce a profit.

***

Most drug companies stopped producing vaccines because vaccines were unprofitable. Arguing that vaccines were necessary, Bill Gates used his fortune to advocate for the transfer of public sector resources to drug companies, so that vaccines, unprofitable under a system of capitalist incentives, would become profitable under a system of government subsidies. Governments would grant exclusive licenses to a few drug companies to manufacture and sell vaccines based on technology developed in publicly-funded government and university labs, while committing to volume purchases of the vaccines. Pharmaceutical firms, in other words, would be granted a license to print money: publicly-funded technology would be handed to them under exclusive licenses and commitments made to pay for bulk purchases. The model was socialist, with one wrinkle. It included generous payouts in interest, dividends and share price appreciation to a parasitic class of coupon clippers, dividend mongers, and stock market gamblers.

Contrary to a popular misconception, socialism doesn't excuse some people from work. Capitalism, however, does. Anyone who lives on drug company securities and share price appreciation is living on the labor of drug company employees and the price-gouging of drug company customers. As for socialism, Lenin invoked a biblical aphorism to explain a fundamental socialist requirement: Those who do not work, shall not eat. Publicly-funded vaccine technology could have been transferred to publicly-owned manufacturers to make vaccines paid for out of the public purse. The only difference would have been that the cost to taxpayers would have been lower because a payout to bond holders and dividend collectors—who contributed nothing to the process that couldn't have been contributed collectively—would have been avoided. In effect, the model Gates proposed amounted to robbery. But then, some would argue that it is on robbery that Gates' fortune is based. He simply proposed a model that had made himself, and other robbers like him, fabulously wealthy.

CHAPTER 6

THE BILLIONAIRE

Who built the seven gates of Thebes?
The books are filled with names of kings.
Was it the kings who hauled the craggy blocks of stone?
— Bertolt Brecht[1]

The billionaire exploits workers and gouges consumers in the
morning, founds charities out of his despoiled wealth in the
afternoon, and receives awards in the evening.[2]

From my point of view, it's more like [the Gates Foundation] are
selling technology than solving problems. — Martin Addo[3]

Let us recognize that our most important contemporaneous
problems are economic and social and not technical
and scientific in the narrow sense that we employ
these words. — Norman Bethune[4]

Bill Gates, billionaire co-founder of the software company Microsoft and the richest person in the world in most years from 1995 to 2017, saw himself as the encephalon of the global response to the Covid-19 pandemic. Gates is the biggest private advocate of vaccines as the principal means of combating infectious diseases and the biggest contributor to the World Health Organization after the United States and Britain. So far as a single-minded focus on vaccines is responsible for the sorry state of the world's pandemic response, Gates bears some responsibility for millions of preventable deaths. For had governments not been so ensorcelled by the idea that vaccines are *the* major way to deal with novel pathogens, they may have taken a page from China's book and implemented a strategy that had actually, demonstrably, worked to shut down Covid-19. Instead, they heeded Gates, a man who has always been obsessed with technology as the sole solution to all problems.

Two days after the World Health Organization declared a pandemic, Gates led a meeting of 12 pharmaceutical executives to plan strategy. He and Fauci, he announced, were "in constant contact."[5] And he was talking with the WHO—always. But he pointed out that "a lot of the work here to stop this epidemic has to do with innovation in diagnostics, therapeutics and vaccines, which isn't really their bailiwick."[6] But it is Gates' bailiwick—or rather, one of his pet projects. Working with the Coalition for Epidemic Preparedness Innovations—a NGO Gates endowed with a $100 million start-up grant to advance the development of vaccines to prepare for epidemics—the billionaire was steering money into Covid-19 vaccine candidates and biotechnologies. In June 2020, the Microsoft co-founder announced that "Every week we're talking with AstraZeneca about, okay, what's going on in India, what's going on in China."[7] According to Tim Schwab, who was following Gates for *The Nation*, the billionaire vaccine activist was presenting himself "as, essentially, leading the global pandemic response."[8] And as Gates acknowledged, the response was "innovation in diagnostics, therapeutics and vaccines," not the non-pharmaceutical public health measures that were in the WHO's bailiwick—the ones that actually worked. Ruling class journalists beat a path to the doors of Gates and Fauci for "expert opinion," when they ought to have been talking to the Chinese.

In 2000, Gates set up a charitable foundation, the Bill and Melinda Gates Foundation, after leading Microsoft for 25 years as chairman and CEO. The foundation's ostensible purpose is to bankroll good works—or what Gates calls good works. The real purpose is to burnish Gates' reputation, which had been tarnished by Microsoft's anti-competitive practices in the 1990s.

Gates has $180 billion at his disposal, including $130 billion in private wealth and $50 billion in his foundation. The foundation is the largest in the world, with assets larger than those of nearly 70 percent of countries. Gates' enormous wealth allows him to buy considerable influence and to promote his point of view in his areas of concern: global health and education.

The foundation has 1,600 employees and employs former pharmaceutical executives in its top ranks, including Dr. Trevor Mundel, formerly global head of development at Novartis, and Emilio Emini, previously senior vice president of vaccine research at Pfizer. The foundation installs its executives on the boards of multiple non-profits; funds academic research; and directly invests in drug companies. It has financial stakes valued at nearly $205 million in nine pharmaceutical companies, including CureVac, Novartis, GlaxoSmithKline, and Sanofi, as well as Gilead, maker of the anti-viral drug Remdesivir; Merck, maker of the antiviral pill, Molnupiravir; and BioNTech, the partner with Pfizer in the manufacturer of the leading mRNA Covid-19 vaccine. The foundation is a major BioNTech shareholder, with a $55 million stake in the company.

Gates claims to use his foundation to put "all the tools of capitalism" to work in order to "connect the promise of philanthropy with the power of private enterprise." In the Gates' view of philanthropy, giving is transformed from donations to the needy to donations to private enterprise to help the needy. He calls this creative capitalism.

Over two decades the Gates Foundation has made close to $2 billion in tax-deductible "charitable" donations to private companies to: develop new drugs; improve sanitation in the developing world; develop financial products for Muslim consumers; and produce news stories about the foundation's work. The beneficiaries, apart from multiple drug companies, have included Unilever, IBM, and NBC Universal Media.

To Gates, the desired role of government is to facilitate the acquisition of fortunes by billionaires, and to create an environment that allows the wealthy to use part of their fortunes to define what social problems ought to be addressed, how the problems are to be understood, and how they are to be solved.

Gates views government as an apparatus to be used by philanthropy, the private sector and civil society to "scale up" whatever philanthropy, i.e., Gates, proposes, rather than as an instrument of its citizens to democratically define what problems are to be addressed and how they are to be solved. The multibillionaire believes his fortune confers upon him a *noblesse oblige* to manage how people think about the issues that affect their lives, what the solutions are, who should implement them, and how.

Gates became interested in vaccines in the late 1990s, at a time Microsoft was facing an antitrust case that cast him as a modern-day robber baron, and he was searching for a pet project he could champion to rehabilitate his sullied public image. In 1998, the US government brought a suit against Microsoft, alleging that it had engaged in anti-competitive behavior to create a monopoly. The court ruled in favor of the government in 1999. Microsoft appealed the decision, and a settlement was reached between the two parties in 2001.

Gates was drawn to vaccine development because it involved creating new technology, Gates' specialty, and because vaccines could be presented as a public good. The billionaire discovered that many Western drug companies had stopped producing vaccines because, as we've seen, immunizations were unprofitable. Gates advocated a new business model involving subsidies, advance market commitments, and volume guarantees. His foundation spent more than $16 billion on vaccine programs, one-quarter going to Gavi, the Global Alliance of Vaccine Initiatives, an NGO Gates helped create to promote immunization programs around the world. Gates' recipe for pandemic preparedness is to create the capability to produce a vaccine in 100 days and manufacture enough doses to immunize the world in the next 100 days. This is precisely the plan announced (copied) by Eric Lander, Joe Biden's science adviser.

Gates uses his billions to set the global health agenda. One way he does so is by buying influence at the World Health Organization. The billionaire's foundation contributed $455 million to the global health body from 2018-2019, making it the organization's third largest contributor after Britain ($464 million) and the United States ($853 million.) The fourth largest funder was Gavi ($389 million), the Gates-led NGO, which had received $4 billion in Gates Foundation injections over two-decades. Gavi leads the WHO's immunization program. Together, the Gates Foundation and Gavi contributed $919 million to the WHO, effectively making Gates the organization's top contributor from 2018-2019. Michele Greenstein and Jeremy Loffredo, writing in the Grayzone, noted that "The sheer magnitude of the foundation's financial contributions to the WHO makes Bill Gates the *de facto* leader at the organization and unelected global health czar."[9] Amir Attaran, a University of Ottawa professor of law and medicine, characterizes the Gates Foundation as, "at best, an adjunct to WHO and at worst a hostile takeover and a usurpation."[10]

Gates' influence over the organization is visible in a number of ways. First, the director-general is a Gates protégé. Before becoming the WHO's leader, Tedros sat on the board of the Gates-founded and -funded Gavi, and was board chair of the Gates-founded and -funded Global Fund to Fight AIDS, Tuberculosis and Malaria. Second, "few policy initiatives or normative standards set by the WHO are announced before they have been casually, unofficially vetted by Gates Foundation staff," according to Laurie Garrett, writing in *Foreign Affairs*.[11] The "Global Vaccine Plan" adopted in 2012 by the World Health Assembly—the decision-making body of the WHO—was co-authored by the Gates Foundation. Third, the Gates Foundation doesn't simply hand over hundreds of millions of dollars every year to the WHO to help the organization carry out its mission; instead, it tells the body what its mission ought to be, and expects compliance with Gates' vision, as a condition of receiving the billionaire's contributions.

The WHO mainly spends Gates Foundation money on polio eradication. Gates has been the world's loudest voice for eradication of polio, and has contributed $1.3 billion to the project. The campaign, begun in 1985, has proved highly successful. Case loads have dropped 99 percent, but success has come at a high price. Some $9 billion has been spent on the project at a cost of about $1 billion per year. By comparison, the campaign to eradicate small pox cost $500 million in today's dollars. Some experts argue that polio is ineradicable, and that continued large expenditures on the effort is a waste of money. They counter that the money invested in the Quixotic effort to completely expunge an ineradicable disease that afflicts few ought to be directed instead to more pressing concerns, such as preventing many millions of deaths from pneumonia, diarrhea, measles, meningitis, and malaria. But Gates insists his contributions can be squandered in whatever fashion he pleases.

Gates uses his billions not only to define which diseases are important, but also how they are to be fought. Fighting malaria with vaccines is another Gates' priority. The billionaire's foundation has invested $1.2 billion in the project.

While we think of malaria as a disease of the global south, it was once present in other parts of the world, including Western Europe and the United States. Indeed, the origins of the Centers for Disease Control and Prevention lie in malaria control. The body was established in 1946 with the primary mission of combating malaria in the swamps and backwoods of the United States, as far north as New Jersey.[12]

Malaria is a disease of underdevelopment. It disappears when development makes environments inhospitable to the pathogen's carriers, mosquitoes. Mosquitoes thrive in stagnant water. When swamps are paved over or drained for agriculture and irrigation canals and dams prevent the pooling of water, mosquito populations diminish. Development also means houses with windows to keep mosquitoes out.

Sardinia, a poor, underdeveloped region of Italy, the largest island in the Mediterranean after Sicily, had long been plagued by malaria. Italian scientists pursued a national antimalarial campaign based on health education, economic development, and treatment of the disease with quinine. After the fall of Mussolini, and with the arrival of US forces in the region, US medicine took over. The Italian campaign was rejected in favor of "the 'American thesis' that malaria could be vanquished by employing technology alone to eradicate mosquitoes, thereby halting the transmission of the disease without the need to address complex social and economic issues." To combat malaria, US scientists, funded by the Rockefeller Foundation, rolled out "the atomic bomb of the insect world": DDT, their "single weapon of choice."[13] Defeating "malaria by means of DDT first in Sardinia and then on a global scale would provide a stunning display of the might of US science and technology," wrote Frank W. Snowden. "The prospect was all the more appealing since US firms such as Du Pont and Monsanto would play a prominent role in supplying DDT. Furthermore, the 'American solution' to the problem of malaria would obviate the need to attend to recalcitrant problems of poverty, land reclamation projects, and environmental degradation. Raising those issues smacked of social medicine and socialism."[14]

The parallel with the "American thesis" that Covid-19 could be vanquished by employing vaccines is revealing. To combat the coronavirus, US scientists, funded by Washington and grants from the Gates Foundation, rolled out the atomic bomb of the viral world: mRNA vaccines, their single weapon of choice. Defeating Covid-19 by means of mRNA vaccines would provide a stunning display of US science and technology. The prospect was all the more appealing since US firms such as Pfizer and Moderna would play a prominent role in supplying inoculations. Furthermore, the "American solution" to the problem would obviate the need to employ non-pharmaceutical public health measures, which smacked of social medicine and the Chinese.

The Gates Foundation's faith in technology as the solution to disease recapitulates the hubris of the period 1945 to the 1990s when "infectious diseases were thought to be easily eradicable." The "prevailing reasoning" wrote Snowden, "held that technology could be counted on to develop weapons of such power as to eliminate communicable diseases one by one."[15]

In the autumn of 2021, GlaxoSmithKline, a pharmaceutical company in which the Gates Foundation has a substantial investment, announced that after 30 years of effort, it had developed an antimalarial vaccine for children, called Mosquirix. The Gates-dominated World Health Organization approved the vaccine, despite reservations about the inoculation's efficacy and practicability.

The vaccine prevented only one-third of severe cases of malaria in young children over a four-year trial period. By contrast, "preventive measures such as bed nets, antimalarials and pesticides ... helped cut deaths from malaria by around 45%."[16] Vaccine uptake is likely to be low. The treatment requires four doses over 18 months. In a test setting in Kenya, only four in 10 eligible infants showed up for their final dose on their second birthday. Between 50 million and 100 million doses will be needed annually by 2030. Billions of dollars will need to be invested in extra production capacity. And yet it's expected that for every 230 children vaccinated, only one will be saved. There is a danger that money spent producing vaccine doses will deplete investment in more effective non-pharmaceutical preventive measures and social medicine. If the danger is realized, Africans will suffer. All the same, GlaxoSmithKline and its major investors—among them, the Gates Foundation—will benefit.

Gates uses his influence over public health agendas to promote new vaccines and therapeutics—pharmaceutical innovation—as the solutions of choice to global health problems. His message is always that "Big Pharma is awesome."[17] In 2014, Gates' then wife Melinda, who was a co-trustee of the foundation along with Bill, said "we believe in the power of innovation to solve problems."[18] Melinda was echoing "the American solution"— the profit-friendly application of US technology to every problem. Gates' gushing over the awesomeness of Big Pharma just might have something to do with the fact that his foundation has a stake in Big Pharma in excess of $200 million.

***

The idea that the Gates Foundation is a charitable organization is misleading. Most people think of charity as giving money to aid an organization that does good works to carry out its mission, not to tell the organization what its mission ought to be and how it should be achieved. What's more, we don't think of contributions that provide a financial return as charity but as investments. The Gates Foundation makes grants to private sector enterprises in which it has financial stakes, and, astonishingly, collects tax benefits in return.

Gates made nearly $250 million in "charitable" grants to drug companies to which his foundation has financial ties, including Merck, Novartis, GlaxoSmithKline, and Sanofi. Consistent with the idea that capitalism is philanthropic and that private enterprise, with the help of philanthropy and government, can solve humanity's ills, the foundation argues that its grants are used for the development of new drugs, that new drugs improve the human condition, and that Gates' grants *cum* investments are therefore philanthropic. From 2016 to 2020, the foundation generated $28.5 billion in investment income, while paying out grants of $23.5 billion.[19] Gates effectively made charitable contributions to himself.

The rewards of Gates' phony philanthropy are munificent and multifarious. Gates claims a reputational benefit, posing as one of humanity's great benefactors. Even Bernie Sanders, who frequently rails against billionaires, views Gates as one of a handful of "great billionaires."[20] Gates uses his contributions to set the agenda of the organizations to which he contributes. None of his contributions are unconditional; they all have strings attached. And he reaps a dual financial reward in the form of returns on his investment and a tax reduction.

***

On top of extolling the awesomeness of Big Pharma, Gates is a vigorous exponent of the strong patent protections upon which Big

Pharma depends for its Big Profits, which it returns in Big Dividends to Big Shareholders like Gates and other Big Billionaires. Gates uses his "philanthropy" "to advance a pro-patent agenda on pharmaceutical drugs, even in countries that are really poor," according to Tim Schwab.[21] This is hardly surprising. Apart from the direct pecuniary interest Gates has in strong patent protection as an investor in scores of enterprises that depend on monopoly pricing laws to legalize their price gouging, Gates' fortune is built on patent protection of Microsoft software. Indeed, Microsoft lobbied strenuously for the 1995 Trade-Related Aspects of Intellectual Property Rights (TRIPS) agreement, that established a global patent regime.

Gates argued that patents should not be lifted on Covid-19 vaccines. If they were, he warned, vaccine makers would fail to recover their research and development costs and would be discouraged from making future investments in new vaccines. This conveniently ignored the massive public sector support Moderna, Pfizer-BioNTech, AstraZeneca, and Johnson & Johnson received in grants, subsidies, and advance purchase agreements—aid that Gates himself argued Big Pharma needed, otherwise vaccine production would not be financially viable.

Gates replied to criticisms of patents as deterrents to the rapid roll-out of vaccines to low- and middle-income countries by noting that "in global health it takes a decade between when a vaccine comes into the rich world and when it gets into the poor countries."[22] Since the roll-out was expected to take less than 10 years, Gates counseled that we rejoice in this faster distribution, even though the lifting of patent protections would accelerate the roll-out even more. The argument was sophistical. It was like telling an employee: "I can pay you $100 per hour, which is the value of what you produce. But I'm only going to pay you $10, and you should be happy with that, because it's twice what I paid you last week." The reality is that lifting patent protections on Covid-19 vaccines would reduce payouts on Gates' investments in BioNTech and other vaccine manufacturers, presumably the reason for his opposition.

In a further effort to torpedo the anti-patent campaign, Gates likened patent waivers to socialism, and intimated that vaccine development was only possible within a capitalist system. "North Korea doesn't have that many vaccines, as far as we can tell," he said.[23] North Korea may not have vaccines (or may—it's difficult to know what the hyper-secretive country does or doesn't have), but Cuba—hardly a capitalist paragon—does have vaccines, and they are home-grown. Indeed, Cuba is a biopharmaceutical leader, with multiple independently developed vaccines, not only for Covid-19, but for a number of other infectious diseases, as well. While North Korea invests in self-defense, allowing the embattled country to develop weapons systems far in advance of any produced by countries of a comparable income level, Cuba invests in biopharmaceuticals—investments that make the country "a biotech juggernaut," according to Gail Reed, the editor of *MEDICC Review*. The socialist country's public health accomplishments are undeniable, she says.[24]

Cuba exports hundreds of millions of vaccines every year to over 40 countries. Of 12 vaccines administered to Cuban children, eight are made domestically. The Communist-led country has eliminated polio, diphtheria, measles, rubella, and whooping cough. Cuba has also developed a lung cancer vaccine, which is undergoing clinical trials at the Roswell Park Comprehensive Cancer Center in New York. The Caribbean country developed two coronavirus vaccines—which don't require extreme refrigeration, as mRNA vaccines do, making them a practical alternative for use in the global south, where expensive refrigeration equipment is not often available. The vaccines are inexpensive to produce, and easy for the socialist country to manufacture at scale.

Cuba's biopharmaceutical achievements are all the more impressive given the country's limited resources. Its GDP per capita is over seven times smaller than that of the United States and its population is only one thirtieth the size of the United States'. What's more, Cuba labors under very trying economic circumstances—the outcome of a decades-long US program to cripple the country economically. That Cuba has accomplished so much, with so little, in the face of such daunting odds, is a refutation of Gates' claim that vaccine and pharmaceutical prowess gestates exclusively in a capitalist womb.

Echoing Gates' nonsense about patent protection, Albert Bourla, chief executive of Pfizer, told an interviewer that, "The only reason why we have vaccines right now was because there was a vibrant private sector. The vibrancy of the private sector, the lifeblood, is the IP protection."[25] What Bourla—who had recently joined Gates in the ranks of billionaires—didn't mention was that his newfound super-wealth is based on technology developed by US government scientists and researchers at the University of Pennsylvania—that is, by the public sector.[26] IP protection allows Bourla and other Pfizer shareholders to monopolize a publicly-funded and -developed invention—that is, to turn a people's vaccine into their private money-making machine. Contrary to Bourla's myth-making, investors were averse to funding companies in their early days that had new ideas about how to make vaccines. Instead, the job fell to the public sector, the only actor prepared to assume the risk, challenging the myth that government is an impediment to free enterprise, rather than its prop.[27]

***

Gates has his fingers in many pies—including in Oxford University's vaccine development program. The program, operating out of the university's Jenner Institute—named after Edward Jenner, the vaccine pioneer who developed the smallpox vaccine—received a $384 million grant from Gates through CEPI. CEPI reflects Gates' thinking that vaccines are the way to fight global outbreaks of communicable diseases. The organization's goal is "to co-ordinate and finance the development of new vaccines for diseases that might lead to a pandemic." It is also "working to create a stockpile of potential treatments for known coronaviruses, hemorrhagic fevers and other global threats that could quickly go into production in the event of an epidemic." On top of funding the Jenner Institute through CEPI, Gates also makes contributions directly from his foundation. The chairman of the Gates Foundation's scientific advisory committee, Sir John Bell, a Canadian-born immunologist, leads the development of Oxford's health research strategies. Just as, in the words of Amir Attaran, the Gates Foundation is at best an adjunct of the WHO, and more likely its conqueror, so too does the foundation bear a similar relationship to the Jenner Institute.

Gates' domination of the institute became evident when the organization's researchers developed a promising viral-vector vaccine against Covid-19. Like most people, they believed vaccines should be public goods, available to all humanity, and not exploited for commercial gain. The inventors offered to issue "nonexclusive, royalty-free licenses" that would allow drug manufacturers to produce the vaccine at low cost. Bell was aghast. He immediately contacted Dr. Trevor Mundel, president of the Gates Foundation's global health division. Mundel got in touch with Gates. Gates got in touch with Oxford. The billionaire persuaded the university to sign an exclusive vaccine deal with the British pharmaceutical giant, AstraZeneca, pressuring the university to give it exclusive rights to the invention and allowing the firm to sell the vaccine at whatever price suited the company's shareholders. Gates has no patience for humanitarians who want to deny the billionaire class attractive money-making opportunities for a project as contemptible as promoting the good of humanity.

For all Gates' self-proclaimed genius, business-savvy, and vaccine expertise, AstraZeneca turned out to be a poor choice. The company had no experience with vaccine development except for a little-known nasal-spray flu vaccine. Its inexperience became evident when it made serious errors in clinical trials. It mixed up dosages. The FDA criticized it for releasing vaccine data that were outdated and potentially misleading. Additionally, the company was plagued by production problems and missed delivery deadlines. Gates had blundered.

***

On a spring day in Finland some four months after the novel coronavirus was identified, virologists at the University of Helsinki were celebrating. They had developed a vaccine to immunize the world against the new viral threat. If it was safe and effective, it would represent a significant advance. Unlike most Covid-19 vaccines under development, which would require an intramuscular injection, their vaccine would be administered nasally, by a spray. This had a number of advantages. The vaccine could be administered quickly and easily. Administration through the nose mobilized an immune response where SARS-CoV-2 infections start. And it wouldn't have to be stored in extremely cold temperatures, as the proposed mRNA vaccines would. Best of all, the researchers wanted to make their invention free to the world—an open source technology—just as the Oxford University scientists had wanted to bestow a gift upon humanity in the form of an open-license vaccine—that is, until "the philanthropist" Bill Gates stopped them. All they had to do was find someone to put up the money to run the clinical trials that would determine whether the vaccine actually had the promise they believed it had.

Finding someone to pay for the clinical trials turned out to be more difficult than the virologists imagined. It's not that no one wanted to back the project; it was just that no one wanted to back development of a vaccine whose inventors insisted it should be shared with the world as a license-free technology. Pharmaceutical companies and venture capitalists won't fund trials for patent-free vaccines. Undaunted, the scientists turned to the Finnish government. Surely, it would put up the money to test a made-at-home vaccine that could save humanity from a virus that, at the time, was killing tens of thousands of people every week around the globe. Their assumption was faulty. The government turned them down. Governments may have lavished munificent assistance on Moderna, Pfizer, BioNTech, Johnson & Johnson, and AstraZeneca, but these firms had their eye on all that matters in capitalist pharmacy: profits. No capitalist government was going to back humanitarian scientists who wanted to give away their intellectual property *gratis* for the benefit of humanity.[28]

***

Having sold the world on the idea that vaccines should be the main tool in the fight against pandemics, Gates now had to sell the world on the view that capitalism would be the best way to deliver vaccine doses to the planet's 7.9 billion inhabitants. The project would be difficult, since a lot of other people didn't share his point of view. And some of those people worked at the World Health Organization.

In March 2020, the WHO created the Covid-19 Technology Access Pool, or C-TAP. The aim of C-TAP was to make the response to Covid-19 a public common good. With humanity facing a shared problem, the best and fastest way, it seemed, to meet the Covid-19 challenge was to pull together. Rather than individual countries, and individual labs, working in isolation, the most promising environment for the rapid development and deployment of technology to combat the coronavirus plague, would be one in which all countries and labs collaborated, sharing ideas, knowledge, research, techniques, and methods, with the common aim of quickly finding solutions to a common problem. The WHO called on the global community to voluntarily deposit research and associated intellectual property to a global knowledge fund for the duration of the pandemic to encourage collaboration and sharing. This, the global health body believed, would enable "multiple manufacturers that currently have untapped capacity to scale up production" of tools to fight the pandemic. The idea was functionally equivalent to the demand made later by South Africa and India, and backed by a number of other countries, to suspend patents on Covid-19 vaccines temporarily, in order to deploy unused manufacturing capacity to the production of generic copies. As it turned out, no major pharmaceutical company shared its technology with C-TAP. And governments took no steps to compel them to do so. C-TAP was a failure.

C-TAP assumed naively that the world would pull together in a common struggle against a common viral enemy simply because it was the right and smart thing to do. It assumed equally naively that private enterprise would voluntarily forgo the opportunity latent in the pandemic to greatly expand its capital by privatizing publicly-developed innovations in vaccines and therapeutics. And it just as naively believed that governments—interlocked in multitudinous ways with the business community and hemmed in by capitalist imperatives—would compel private enterprise to do what was right for humanity rather than what was right for private enterprise. All the same, the idea that the normal rules of business had to be suspended if humanity was to vanquish the menace of Covid-19 had traction, and something had to be done about it. Capitalism, in the Gates' view, wasn't the problem.

One month after the WHO called upon the global community to voluntarily share intellectual property (i.e., to waive patent protections for the duration of the pandemic), Gates counterpunched with the Access to Covid Tools-Accelerator, or ACT-A. Launched by the WHO, the European Commission, France, and the Gates Foundation, the accelerator was, despite the presence of other sponsors, a Gates' operation through and through; it was designed, managed, and staffed largely by the foundation's employees. Its mandate was "to accelerate the development, production, and equitable access to COVID-19 tests, treatments, and vaccines." The accelerator's vaccine arm—which would work on getting shots into arms quickly —would be run by three Gates-dominated organizations—Gavi, as the lead, and CEPI and the WHO, as partners. UNICEF would lead delivery efforts. ACT-A's vaccine arm would be named COVAX.

The thinking behind COVAX was simple. Vaccines needed to be developed and manufactured quickly and distributed equitably. COVAX would leave patent protections in place, so that a few vaccine makers could divide the world market among themselves, returning hefty dividends to their shareholders, among them, Gates himself. COVAX would act as the vaccine purchasing agent for the world. The rich countries would transfer funds to the facility, which would then buy vaccines for everyone, including 92 poor countries, which would receive vaccine doses *gratis*. In this way, every contributor would pay the same price, and vaccines could be distributed equitably from the COVAX repository in proportion to population and not according to ability to pay.

COVAX was a feint toward a communist-style each-according-to-their-need vaccine distribution system. The impetus, however, was not humanitarianism, but saving intellectual property protection from efforts to temporarily suspend it. COVAX failed in its communist-style distribution. Rich countries didn't use the facility as a global purchasing agent, preferring instead to make vaccine purchases outside the COVAX facility. Washington paid $11 billion to six vaccine manufacturers for priority access to 600 million doses, with options for millions more. Canada bought doses in quantities multiple times in excess of its own population. Seeing where the game was headed, 17 countries eligible for free COVAX doses made individual deals with vaccine manufacturers. What's more, COVAX depended heavily on the Serum Institute, the giant Indian vaccine manufacturer, to produce hundreds of millions of doses to be shared around the world. Those plans were scotched when the Indian government, reeling under an escalating Covid-19 crisis, banned the company from exporting vaccine doses so that the firm's manufacturing capacity could be monopolized for domestic production. With the world's rich countries, and some of the poor, seeking doses outside of COVAX, the facility's role as a global purchasing agent collapsed. In the end, COVAX became a mechanism for providing vaccine aid to poor countries that couldn't afford to compete for doses on the open market.

Additionally, COVAX failed to quell demands for the lifting of patent protections; those demands continued, especially after it became evident that the rich countries had cleared the shelves, leaving the world's poor without access to inoculations. Africa was particularly disadvantaged. Long after most people in the global north were fully vaccinated, the vast majority of Africans still had not received even a single dose. The distribution of vaccines to poor countries was delayed further when the rich countries reinvigorated their monopolization of vaccine doses by buying doses for booster shots, despite two-shot vaccine regimens continuing to provide protection against severe disease and hospitalization. The WHO objected that the rich countries' unnecessary booster gambit not only exacerbated a vaccine apartheid but encouraged the development of more transmissible or virulent variants by allowing the virus to circulate in the global south unchecked by mass immunization. The WHO's fears were borne out when the Omicron variant emerged in Botswana, capable of spreading even more rapidly than the Delta variant, which, itself, was more transmissible than its antecedents. The West's response to the Omicron development was to double down on its booster strategy, which, in large measure, had been the cause of Omicron's emergence.

**

Being wealthy "evidently conveys expertise, at least according to US news media," remarked James Love, an expert on intellectual property. "If we're talking about Gates—he's an expert on malaria, he's an expert on public education, now he's an expert on vaccines."[29] Of course, Gates is neither an expert on education, infectious diseases, or vaccines. But he is an expert on using means legal, illegal, and somewhere in between, to exploit employees and consumers for private gain. He is also, it seems, an expert on how to get the news media to present Bill Gates as an expert in whatever field Bill Gates claims expertise.

Using both his personal fortune and his foundation's endowment, Gates spends liberally on public relations and buys favorable media coverage by making generous grants to media organizations. In the first decade of the twenty-first century, the Gates Foundation spent $1 billion on what it called "advocacy and policy"—about $100 million annually. Advocacy is public relations, a term of obfuscation used to refer to the shaping of public opinion, propaganda, and manufacturing consent. Gates Foundation advocacy is aimed at shaping public opinion to comport with Gates' interests and his view that capitalism is philanthropic and that private enterprise, assisted by government and philanthropy, can solve humanity's problems.

Gates has provided over $300 million in grants to news organizations, including BBC, NBC, Al Jazeera, ProPublica, *The National Journal*, *The Guardian*, Univision, Medium, *The Financial Times*, *The Atlantic*, *The Texas Tribune*, Gannett, *The Washington Monthly*, *Le Monde*, and the Center for Investigative Reporting.[30] The grants, usually tied to Gates' pet projects of global health and education, help elevate his agenda and communicate his point of view to a mass audience. If Gates believes vaccines are the main tool for fighting pandemics, then news media are happy to provide him and his ideas a platform, in return for his generous contributions.

In furtherance of Gates' interests and those of his class, the Gates Foundation funds research on how to manipulate public opinion; gives money to magazines and scientific journals to publish research and articles on topics of interest to the foundation which support Gates' point of view; pays think tanks to produce media fact sheets and newspaper opinion pieces to echo Gates' thinking; backs programs to coach Gates-friendly experts to write columns for media outlets, such as *The New York Times* and *The Huffington Post*; and invests in training journalists to write on issues it cares about in ways that advance Gates' agenda.

Gates' investments in shaping public opinion and manipulating news media have multiple goals: First, to transform his reputation as a modern day robber baron who used illegal means and anti-competitive practices to accumulate a vast fortune into a selfless sponsor of good works, a visionary leader in the fields of global health and education, an expert on vaccines, malaria, and pandemics, and a savior of humanity; second, to transform the reality that the activities of the Gates Foundation are self-serving into the fiction that they are philanthropic; to promote the idea that capitalism is philanthropic and that humanity's ills are best solved by private enterprise; to define what the most pressing global health problems are and then to promote Big Pharma as the solution; and to defend intellectual property protection. As a consequence of

Gates' investments in public relations and the media, not only does Gates become the subject of news media puff pieces and glowing editorials; not only do media outlets portray him as the world's health czar and point person on the global response to the Covid-19 crisis; but his agenda and points of view are brought to the fore of public attention. If the view of most of the world's governments is that the route to addressing the Covid-19 pandemic is vaccines (rather than a combination of non-pharmaceutical public health measures and safe and effective inoculations), it is largely because Gates has spent hundreds of millions of dollars on advocacy to make this view the common sense of the age.

***

Bill Gates' enormous wealth allows the billionaire to buy enormous influence. He sets research, public policy, and media agendas by carefully doling out largesse to individuals and organizations that help advance his aims. Moreover, by labelling his investments as philanthropy, Gates inveigles the public to subsidize his self-serving efforts. That's because Gates receives a tax benefit whenever he uses "philanthropy" to advance his own interests. In this way, philanthropic foundations, like Gates', displace tax revenue. And while it might be thought that as a condition of receiving tax breaks that billionaires must prove that their charitable contributions are indeed charitable, that's not the case. The estimated cost to the US Treasury of the billionaire class's practice of making phony charitable contributions to causes, organizations, and enterprises that protect and promote its interests is $40 billion, according to former US labor secretary and economist Robert B. Reich.[31] It's a scam, organized by the billionaire class's best friend—the US Congress.

Gates provides largesse to organizations that lobby for industry-friendly government policies and regulation, such as the Drug Information Association, directed by Big Pharma. He showers money upon think tanks and advocacy groups that want to prevent government from intervening in the economy on behalf of ordinary people and the employee class. He also directs "philanthropic" resources to lobby groups that help promote business's agenda *contra* working class interests, such as the American Enterprise Institute, which has received nearly $7 billion in Gates' "charity," and the US Chamber of Commerce, which Gates has favored with over $15 million in "philanthropic" contributions. Gates, like other billionaires, uses his wealth to persuade governments to implement policies that benefit his business interests, and receives a tax deduction in return as an ancillary benefit.

Gates cheats the public in four ways. (1) He has amassed his wealth partly through monopoly pricing, charging consumers more for Microsoft products than they would have paid had his company not engaged in anti-competitive practices. (2) His vast wealth is the product of paying hundreds of thousands of employees less than the value of what they produced. (3) The tax credits he receives for his spurious philanthropy increase the amount of taxes the public must bear to compensate for the credits he receives. (4) His "philanthropy" is directed toward the promotion of programs and policies, such as the protection of intellectual property, and capitalist pseudo-solutions to pressing problems, that line the pockets of billionaires at the expense of the public.

Gates' fortune was not produced by Bill himself; he only accumulated it. It was produced collectively by numberless people, backed by public funds and public sector inventions. The decisions over how collectively-produced wealth is used ought to be made collectively, by the people who produced and helped produce it. Instead, Gates' fortune, and the Gates Foundation endowment, is used in whatever way Bill alone chooses. He has chosen to use his accumulated wealth to line his pockets, investing it under the guise of charity in firms in which he has a financial stake, and to set agendas which advance his individual and class interests. Bill Gates is concealing self-promotion, agenda setting, fortune building, and the whitewashing of capitalism behind philanthropy, and through this deception has maneuvered the public into subsidizing his activities through the tax benefits his phony charitable contributions allow him to claim. He is capitalism personified: equal parts parasite and fraudster.

***

If the early English capitalist state was distinguished by its ability to take pounds out of taxpayers' pockets to put sailors on the open sea and soldiers in the field—all in the service of the burgeoning English bourgeoisie's overseas interests—then in the face of a twenty-first century global public health emergency, the US state distinguished itself by its ability to take dollars out of taxpayers' pockets to place dividends in the pockets of Big Pharma shareholders by putting vaccines in people's arms. Make no mistake: Washington—which is to say, US taxpayers—bankrolled the vaccines that protect many of us from serious illness and hospitalization. Covid-19 vaccines are the product of Big Government, not Big Pharma.

The United States, the European Union, Britain, Russia, and China played major roles in developing Covid-19 vaccines. Governments spent billions of dollars to: acquire raw materials for manufacturers; fund their clinical trials; furnish their factories with equipment; and guarantee purchases of their finished product. On top of that, governments financed the basic research on which new—and even old—vaccine technologies were based. Pfizer licensed technology developed at the University of Pennsylvania and in US government labs through its partner BioNTech. Moderna capitalized on University of Pennsylvania research and collaborated with the National Institutes of Health to develop its vaccine (which the NIH called the NIH-Moderna vaccine and Fauci claimed was developed solely by government scientists and not co-invented by Moderna).[32] AstraZeneca licensed technology developed by researchers at Oxford University. Russian scientists tapped into strengths in virology and vaccines from the Soviet era, when the USSR was the world leader in these disciplines.

In the United States, central planning of vaccine production was taken on by Operation Warp Speed (OWS). Washington recognized that the development and manufacture of Covid-19 vaccines was beyond the risk tolerance of private industry. Most vaccine prospects fail, and historically, successful shots took years to develop, at considerable cost. Large investments in clinical trials would be required, and the significant expense would be for nought if a safe and effective vaccine could not be found, as it seemed would likely happen. After all, despite decades of effort, an AIDS vaccine had yet to be developed. Additionally, an effective vaccine might have adverse side-effects, creating costly legal troubles. And what if the Covid-19 pandemic burned itself out before a vaccine could be brought to market? Finally, because Covid-19 vaccines would be seen as a public good, the companies' latitude in pricing would be limited by public policy concerns rather than guided by shareholder value considerations. Better to focus resources on developing the kind of drugs capitalist imperatives compelled the pharmaceutical industry to develop: blockbusters that would manage, not cure, the chronic conditions of affluent consumers in rich countries.

Big Pharma leaned toward patentable pills that were inexpensive to produce, that patients would have to take for a lifetime, and that could be priced well above cost. From an investor perspective, diverting resources from the search for the next blockbuster to developing vaccines for a pandemic that might peter out, was just dumb. "Private companies can't take that kind of risk," Gates observed.[33] But governments can. If capitalist incentives prevented the private sector from taking on the job, then government would have to step in. Or, to put it another way, if capitalist incentives prevented the private sector from doing the job, capitalist domination of the state meant that governments would be used to turn an unprofitable activity into a highly profitable opportunity.

Operation Warp Speed was the kind of operation Gates had been advocating for years. Despite the myth that capitalism, in its alleged philanthropic way, will eventually solve all problems, there are plenty of problems the private sector won't touch. Covid-19 was one of them. But to Gates' thinking, private enterprise could be used to solve problems if governments and philanthropists made it worth its while. This could be done by paying companies to work on solving difficult problems—like, say, malaria, or improving student test scores, or making a vaccine to fight a new virus. Private enterprise, if successful, could sign hosannas to itself, while Gates extolled capitalism and cashed in on his investments in the recipients of public largesse.

Operation Warp Speed "took nearly all the risk away from private pharmaceutical companies,"[34] remarked Scott Atlas, who for a time was a Trump Covid-19 adviser. Conceived by Dr. Peter Marks, the Food and Drug Administration's top vaccine regulator, OWS would be a collaboration between the US military, which would look after logistics, and the Department of Health and Human Services, which would handle planning. OWS planning was headed by pharmaceutical industry executives, whose first important role was to select the companies that would be invited to suckle at Lady Liberty's teat. Despite the obvious conflict of interest, the executives were granted special exemptions to keep their financial stakes in the companies they were making decisions about.

The OWS supremo, Moncef Slaoui, was a Big Pharma executive who had spent 30 years at GlaxoSmithKline (GSK), where he had eventually headed its R&D department. Slaoui had $10 million in GSK stock holdings. He also had over $12 million in Moderna shares and had been on the company's board since 2017. Slaoui resigned from the company's board when he joined OWS, but kept over $10 million in stock options.

Slaoui reported to Alex M. Azar II, the health and human services secretary, who had spent three years as president of Eli Lilly's US subsidiary. Pfizer executives William Erhardt and Rachel Harrigan were brought on board as advisers. Both were allowed to retain their financial stakes in Pfizer.

OWS chose six companies from 50 vaccine candidates. In order to maximize the chance that at least one of them would succeed, Slaoui and his team decided to pick two companies from each of three different vaccine platforms. These would be mRNA (Moderna and Pfizer-BioNTech); viral vector (AstraZeneca and Johnson & Johnson); and protein-based (Novavax and Sanofi/GSK).

After Slaoui's team chose Moderna, the company's share price soared. Two weeks later, Slaoui received options to buy a further 18,270 shares. Erhardt's and Harrigan's employer, Pfizer, was granted a guaranteed purchase order of $1.95 billion.

Taxpayer money would flow "to a small group of capitalists with almost no strings attached and little transparency,"[35] Nina Burleigh observed. OWS ensured the US government would cover the cost of development, guide the clinical trials, and deliver supplies to factories. It would also guarantee payment for doses, even if development efforts failed to pan out.

The US government financed Moderna's clinical trials at a cost of $900 million. It also gifted the company with $3.2 billion in advanced purchase orders, topped up with $2.5 billion to buy raw materials, expand its factory, and hire more employees. AstraZeneca received $1.2 billion from Washington and $79 million from London for vaccines, and a further $486 million from the United States to produce a monoclonal antibody drug. Johnson & Johnson received $500,000 in US funding. Novavax got $1.6 billion, while Pfizer-BioNTech got 400 million euros from Germany, $120 million from the European Investment Bank, and $1.95 billion in an advance purchase contract from Washington. Pfizer called on Washington multiple times to get access to manufacturing supplies. Merck received $105 million in US government funding to make vaccines for Johnson & Johnson, along with $29 million and $1.2 billion in advance purchase orders to develop an antiviral pill, while Washington gave Regeneron $450 million for therapeutics. Meanwhile, Sanofi/GSK netted a cool $2.1 billion from Uncle Sam.

Pfizer-BioNTech and Moderna turned out to be the big winners. Their mRNA vaccines grew to be widely regarded as the *nec plus ultra* of Covid-19 inoculations. Significantly, although not surprisingly, an anonymous US government scientist was largely responsible for the success of the companies' vaccines. Barney Graham "specialized in the kind of long, expensive research that only governments bankroll,"[36] *The Wall Street Journal* explained. In 2016, while working on a vaccine against MERS, Graham developed a method to bioengineer a viral protein that could be used to develop vaccines. BioNTech, Pfizer's partner, licensed the technique. Graham started working with Moderna in 2017 to develop a way to rapidly manufacture vaccines, based on his method. When the genetic code of the novel coronavirus was published in January 2020, Graham immediately applied his invention to SARS-Cov-2, and sent instructions to Moderna on how to manufacture a vaccine to target the virus's spike protein. Fauci approved a partnership between Moderna and government scientists, telling them, "Go for it. Whatever it costs, don't worry about it." [37]

Graham's work developed out of a long line of earlier work carried out in publicly funded labs. The idea of encasing drugs or vaccines in a lipid nanoparticle shell originated in the 1960s in the MIT lab of Robert Langer. Two researchers, Drew Weissman and Katalin Kariko, at the University of Pennsylvania, took the idea further. Both BioNTech and Moderna licensed the duo's invention. The two scientists' work also paved the way for Graham. The culmination of the social process of publicly-funded scientists building on the work of other publicly-funded scientists was the Pfizer-BioNTech and Moderna vaccines. The National Institutes of Health, much to Moderna's chagrin, labelled Moderna's vaccine, the NIH-Moderna vaccine, to reflect the significant US government contribution. Fauci averred that the "vaccine was actually developed in my institute's vaccine research center by a team of scientists led by Dr. Barney Graham and his close colleague, Dr. Kizzmekia Corbett."[38] Moderna, seeking to claim an exclusive patent, contested Fauci's claim, insisting its own scientists had independently developed the inoculation. But it was clear that without the intervention of the capitalist state, the vaccine Moderna mendaciously claimed as its own, would never have been developed. Biden officials were "privately adamant," reported *The Washington Post*, that Moderna owed "its success to the US government."[39] It was only one of a multitude of companies about which the same could be said.

CHAPTER 7

THE HENCHMAN

*Capitalism was only interested in the protection of public
health in so far as this was necessary for its own safety.*
— N. Bukharin and E. Preobrazhensky[1]

In the early months of 2020, decision-makers around the world
considered three possible answers to the question of how the pandemic could be brought to an end.

The first answer was to allow the virus to spread until most of
us acquired immunity through infection. If the virus was allowed
to replicate unchecked, a profound economic chaos would ensue,
on top of a large number of deaths. If the spread of the virus was
controlled, economic chaos would be avoided, but the number of
deaths would be just as large, with the difference that the accumulation of fatalities would be distributed over a prolonged period.
Economic upheaval would occur, but rather than being profound
and acute, it would be protracted but mitigated.

The second answer was to vaccinate the world's population,
until most of us acquired vaccine-induced immunity. This had the
advantage of producing community protection without producing a
massive death toll. The problem was that from the coign of vantage
of early 2020, the chances of this approach paying off were slim. It's
not always, or even often, possible to produce vaccines that work,

that are safe, and can be tested, manufactured, and distributed quickly. Prior to 2020, the fastest a vaccine had ever been developed was four years. While we now know that effective vaccines against the novel coronavirus were produced quickly, decision-makers didn't know that vaccines could be produced quickly when the pandemic first hit.

The third answer was to eliminate circulation of the virus through non-pharmaceutical public health measures, including stringent border restrictions. While this worked in China and a few other countries, border restrictions would need to be maintained indefinitely unless the strategy was universally implemented. The chance of every country working in concert to eliminate the virus through non-pharmaceutical public health measures was vanishingly small. And while in principle tough border restrictions could be maintained indefinitely, there would be no foreseeable end to the disruption of a country's economic life that border restrictions would engender.

Of superpowers, the United States and Russia saw the first (mitigation) and second (vaccines) as the most compelling answers to the Covid-19 conundrum. Britain, and most of the middle- and high-income countries shared this view. China opted for the third (elimination) while working on its own vaccines. A small minority of mid- to high-income countries emulated China, adopting the elimination strategy. Rather than using resources to buy their way to the front of the vaccine queue, as Israel and Canada did, these countries invested in robust test, trace, and isolate programs, with the consequence that they held infection and fatality levels to remarkably low levels. But by choosing to invest in a zero-Covid approach, they forfeited the resources they needed to source vaccines rapidly. As a result, they were slower than many other countries to roll out immunizations.

Based on their approach to the pandemic, countries fell into one of four categories:

(1) Mid- to high-income countries that followed a vaccine-centric approach. They saw vaccines as the exit ramp from the pandemic and rushed to get their populations immunized, accepting mitigation as a necessary evil until a vaccine was available.

(2) Mid- to high-income countries that followed an elimination-centric approach. These countries focused on eliminating community transmission, accepting a slower vaccine roll-out as a trade-off.

(3) China. It vigorously pursued elimination while at the same time developing vaccines.

(4) Low-income countries. With the exception of Cuba and Vietnam, low-income countries were neither elimination- nor vaccine-centric. The nature of their economies, with a high degree of informal employment, and their complete dependency on aid to acquire vaccines, ruled out either elimination or rapid vaccine roll-out as feasible options. Cuba and Vietnam initially pursued elimination strategies, but under economic pressure, relaxed their border restrictions, and were soon beset by imported outbreaks. These outbreaks, however, produced infections and mortality per million well below US levels. Cuba, alone among low-income countries, produced Covid-19 vaccines, which were used to inoculate its own population, and for export to allies. North Korea, as we've seen, took the virus "hyper-seriously" and quickly closed its borders. Its claims to have experienced zero cases may, in fact, be true.

**

While the vaccine-centric approach became the approach adopted by decision-makers in most of the mid- to high-income countries, there were plenty of reasons why it should have been regarded with extreme skepticism, and indeed was within the scientific community.

Throughout the first half of 2020 and into the summer of that year, there were serious doubts about whether humans could develop a durable immunity to the novel coronavirus. There are four coronaviruses that produce the common cold, against which no vaccine had ever been developed. "What we know from 60 years of research into these viruses is that they come back year after year and reinfect the same people—over and over again,"[2] observed CNN's William Haseltine. If the novel coronavirus was like coronavirus common colds, it was an open question whether a vaccine effort could ever succeed. The World Health Organization reminded governments that the question of whether humans could acquire immunity to the virus had yet to be answered. As late as October 2020, the British medical journal, The Lancet, would report that "there is no evidence for lasting protective immunity to SARS-CoV-2 following natural infection."[3] Vaccine proponent Anthony Fauci expressed concern. When "you look at the history of the common coronaviruses that cause the common cold, the reports in the literature are that the durability of immunity that's protective ranges from 3 to 6 months to almost always less than a year."[4] Fauci was optimistic that humans could acquire immunity, but pointed out that immune response was only a necessary, not a sufficient, condition of vaccine success. There's "never a guarantee, ever, that you're going to get an effective vaccine,"[5] he warned.

The state of the art in vaccine development in early 2020, when decisions were being made about how to tackle Covid-19, was that almost all vaccine efforts failed. Only 6 percent succeeded.[6] And the very few that did succeed took a long time to come to fruition. The thinking, at that point, was that a new vaccine would likely take between 10 and 15 years to develop. "All the other major vaccines we have—for measles, Ebola—have taken a minimum of seven years, and some as long as 40 years," remarked immunologist James Hildreth.[7] Of the 6 percent of vaccine efforts that did succeed, the average development time was 10.7 years.

Scientists saw little chance a Covid-19 vaccine would be quickly developed. "What people don't realize is that normally vaccine development takes many years, sometimes decades," virologist Dan Barouch told The New York Times.[8] Robert Van Exan, a veteran of the US vaccine industry, assessed the probability of a safe and effective Covid-19 vaccine as "relatively low."[9] The consensus among scientists was that a vaccine, if it arrived, wouldn't arrive soon. Even a few White House officials were skeptical. Some, reported *The Wall Street Journal*, were "trying to talk the president down," arguing that his expectation that an effective vaccine could be produced in record time was unreasonable.[10] Indeed, anyone reviewing the state of the art in 2020 would have reasonably concluded that the chance of a vaccine being rapidly developed was poor. Which raises the question: If vaccine success appeared to be unlikely, and non-pharmaceutical public health measures had already been shown to be effective in curbing the spread of the virus, why were billions of dollars invested in a project that looked like it was almost certain to fail, while at the same time, a demonstrably effective solution to the crisis was rejected?

Ruling class journalist David "Scoop" Sanger raised doubts about whether a vaccine was possible, while at the same time pointing to another concern: safety. The "whole enterprise," he wrote "remains dogged by uncertainty about whether any coronavirus vaccine will prove effective, how fast it could be made available to millions or billions of people and whether the rush—compressing a process that can take 10 years into 10 months—will sacrifice safety."[11] The answer, it turned out, was that safety was sacrificed. Indeed, it was only by sacrificing safety that vaccines were produced quickly. Because "of the pandemic's urgency, any promising Covid-19 vaccine is likely to be fast-tracked through the testing and approval process," he warned. "It may not go through years of clinical trials and careful studies of possible long-term side effects, the way other drugs do."[12] As Sanger predicted, the vaccines were rushed into people's arms before clinical trials were completed and before sufficient time had elapsed to evaluate possible long-term side effects.

The pessimism of the scientists who predicted in 2020 that a vaccine could not possibly be produced in 12 to 18 months can be forgiven. They were assuming that like other vaccines, a Covid-19 vaccine would require a period of testing over many years.

For example, Walter Orenstein, associate director of the Emory Vaccine Center in Atlanta, told *The Wall Street Journal* that he was "skeptical a safe and effective vaccine could be available soon, given all the testing required."[13] What he didn't know was that all the testing required wouldn't be done. Had normal testing protocols been followed, it would have taken two years or more to develop a Covid-19 vaccine, and safe vaccines may never have been developed. (Had trials lasted their planned two years, they may have uncovered mid- to long-term safety concerns that would have ruled out authorization of the shots.)

Normally, vaccines are tested in non-human animals first and then undergo three phases of testing, called clinical trials, in humans. Phase 1 human testing involves trials with a small number of people to determine whether the vaccine produces obvious harm. Trials typically last several months. If the vaccine is found to produce no obvious harm, phase 2 begins. Phase 2 trials involve larger numbers of volunteers. Again, the goal is to screen out vaccines that are manifestly dangerous. Additionally, phase 2 trials look at the question of immunogenicity—assessed *in vitro* through blood tests to determine whether a vaccine provokes an immune response. Phase 2 trials last from several months to two years. If the vaccine seems safe and there is sufficient evidence of immunogenicity, researchers proceed to phase 3. In phase 3, a large number of volunteers is recruited. They are randomly assigned to one of two groups: a vaccine group, in which subjects receive the vaccine; and a placebo group, in which volunteers receive a dummy injection. The two groups are tracked over a period of one to four years. If the rate of infection, hospitalization, and mortality is better in the vaccine group, the vaccine is judged to be effective. At the same time, careful records of side-effects are kept, to evaluate safety.

The phase 3 trials for vaccine candidates selected by Operation Warp Speed lasted only two months before regulators were asked to authorize emergency use of the vaccines. At that point, the vaccine makers had collected enough evidence to show that the trial subjects who received vaccines were less likely than placebo recipients to test positive for Covid-19. However, given that only two months had elapsed, they had insufficient time to assess whether the vaccines were safe over the mid to long term. Despite minimal safety data, the vaccine makers, invoking a "desperate times justify desperate measures" argument, reasoning that the pandemic was a medical emergency and that a medical emergency justified use of vaccines even if the vaccines' safety profile was largely unknown. And since the global bellwether regulator, the US Food and Drug Administration, said it would authorize the use of the vaccines because there were "no adequate, approved, and available alternatives," other regulators followed. However, there *was* an adequate, demonstrably successful and safe, available alternative: the elimination strategy.

Once the regulators authorized vaccine use, the phase 3 trials were effectively brought to a close. One of the troubling implications for volunteers who received a placebo was that they would be left unprotected if they remained in the trials. That wouldn't be an issue if the trials were run in countries that had eliminated community transmission. In these countries, anyone who received a placebo would have had little chance of becoming ill, and therefore it would be impossible to discover whether the vaccine provided protection against illness. For this reason, the trials were conducted in countries with significant outbreaks. Understandably, volunteers in these countries wanted to receive vaccines to protect themselves. The drug companies acceded to their request, effectively ejecting placebo group participants from their trials. This meant that the volunteers who remained in the trials were preponderantly vaccine recipients. Without a placebo group for comparison, safety and efficacy questions could no longer be answered with any degree of certainty.

Anticipating that testing protocols would be circumvented in the rush to get shots into people's arms, Sandra Crouse Quinn, a professor of public health at the University of Maryland, told *The New York Times* that "if you're smart, you're worried that maybe we've moved so fast that we'll accept a level of risk that we might not ordinarily accept."[14] The Chinese Communist Party's newspaper, *Global Times*, thought there were further grounds for concern. Operation Warp Speed's vaccines were based on new technologies. Given that nothing was known about the effects of these technologies on human health, extra caution needed to be taken to protect the billions of people who would be exposed to them. *Global Times* assessed that authorizing the use of experimental technologies before their safety and efficacy had been fully evaluated amounted to "a continuous process of large-scale testing on human beings," which, given that clinical trials had been effectively cut short after only two months, it surely was.[15]

Based on the history of vaccinology, there was reason to believe that the new technologies might produce harm that would only come to light later, especially considering that research, development, and testing protocols had been bypassed in a rush to get vaccines into people's arms. For "virtually every vaccine ever made, the first vaccines aren't always the best, safest, and last," warned Paul A. Offit, a professor of vaccinology at the University of Pennsylvania and co-inventor of the rotavirus vaccine.

> For example, a live, weakened polio vaccine introduced in 1963 was replaced by an inactivated polio vaccine in 2000, when it became clear that the former actually caused polio in eight to ten US children every year. The first measles vaccines in 1963—which caused a high rate of fever and rash—was replaced by a safer, better vaccine in 1968.[16]

Offit saw the development of the Moderna, Pfizer-BioNTech, and AstraZeneca vaccines as "accompanied by a disturbing show of hubris" and "bold pronouncements" that "ignored the likely surprises that lay ahead."[17]

Another measles vaccine, which was introduced in 1963, was taken off the market when it was found to actually increase the risk of pneumonia. The first rubella (German measles) vaccine in 1969, which caused arthritis in small joints like fingers and wrists, was replaced by a safer vaccine in 1979.

The vaccine-makers knew that surprises may lay ahead, and therefore insisted they be granted immunity from any harm their fast-tracked vaccines caused. Johnson & Johnson's Chief Scientific Officer Paul Stoffels told *The Wall Street Journal* that the industry needed liability protection, otherwise it wouldn't produce the vaccines that were needed.[18] The newspaper published Stoffels' comment under a foreboding headline: "People Harmed by Coronavirus Vaccines Will Have Little Recourse." Two mechanisms shielded the drug companies from liability if their Covid-19 vaccines caused sickness or death.[19] The first was US legislation, passed in March, 2020, granting immunity from liability to any commercial enterprise that produced or distributed Covid-19 vaccines.[20] This was buttressed by protection against liability granted to manufacturers who made or distributed vaccines under emergency use authorization. Concern that fast-tracking vaccines meant we were accepting a level of risk that might not ordinarily be accepted was only heightened, then, by the reality that vaccine-makers refused to accept liability for their vaccines and were excused of liability by Washington. This was an implicit recognition that the industry and government worried that vaccine safety hazards might lurk over the horizon. More worryingly, the granting of liability immunity to the industry meant that vaccine-makers could proceed incautiously, knowing they were shielded from penalty.

Once the no-liability model was established in the United States, it was applied across the board in other countries.

As mentioned, after two months of planned two-year phase 3 clinical trials, the vaccine-makers had demonstrated that trial participants who received vaccines were less likely to test positive for Covid-19 than were those who received placebo injections. But they didn't show "whether covid-19 vaccines reduce[d] the risk of hospital admission, intensive care unit admission, severe covid-19, and mortality, as well as whether the vaccines [were] effective in populations at high risk of severe covid-19," including "older, chronically ill, or immunocompromised people, [who] were under-represented in or excluded from trials," reported the *British Medical Journal.*[21]

Also missing were "long term safety data," as well as data on "uncommon adverse events ... risk of vaccine associated enhanced disease; effects in pregnant and breastfeeding women, people who were immunocompromised, frail, or with comorbidities or auto-immune or inflammatory disorders; [and] potential interaction between different vaccines."[22]

The vaccine manufacturers were ordered to conduct studies to fill in the blanks as a condition of authorization. However, rather than producing "data on hard outcomes such as hospital and intensive care admissions or death in moderate or high risk populations" they conducted studies "aimed at developing new vaccines or obtaining approval for additional doses of the current vaccines."[23]

The *British Medical Journal* noted that there was "a long history of concerns ... about the wisdom of shifting clinically important efficacy and safety assessments from before to after authorisation." Often studies were never started, many took years longer than planned, and some failed to confirm pre-authorisation results. Moreover, regulators "only rarely sanction[ed] companies for not adhering to post-authorization study requirements, and drugs [were] only rarely withdrawn."[24]

In sum, Covid-19 vaccines were authorized for use on the basis of minimal safety and efficacy data, on the condition that manufacturers conduct studies after authorization to fill in the blanks—that is, after billions of people had already been exposed to the inoculations. Little, then, was known about the vaccines when they were authorized, and much remains unknown about them today. Not only did decision-makers gamble that a vaccine could be produced in record time, they gambled with the safety of billions of people when they authorized shots about which only the most minimal safety and efficacy data had been collected. It is not unreasonable to think that after enjoying a bonanza of profits, and with the prospect of additional billions of dollars in profits ahead of them, the vaccine-makers would be averse to carrying out studies that could possibly show their vaccines were minimally effective and had inflicted long-term harm on billions of people. And what would regulators do with this information, assuming improbably that the vaccine-makers actually produced it? Recalling vaccines after they have been widely used (and possibly after having caused great harm) would be pointless. In short, Big Pharma was given near *carte blanche* to gamble with the health of billions of people, to address a medical emergency that could have been prevented, had governments simply followed old school pubic health methods as China and a handful of other countries did.

Once the phase 3 trials were effectively abandoned, the drug companies transitioned to non-clinical, uncontrolled, observational studies, comparing those who chose to be vaccinated with those who did not. These studies found that the difference in the rate of infection between these two groups was narrowing. There were two possible explanations: (1) The efficacy of the vaccines was waning. (2) Unvaccinated people as a group were increasingly acquiring natural immunity through infection, and were therefore growing to resemble the vaccinated population in their degree of immunity. Alternatively, or additionally, the vaccinated were taking fewer precautions against infection than they had prior to vaccination, assuming erroneously that the vaccines were 100 percent effective against infection. The vaccine manufacturers, ruling class journalists, and most governments, embraced the first explanation. If vaccine efficacy was waning, it could be argued that booster shots were necessary, and additional revenue streams for Pfizer-BioNTech, Moderna, and other vaccine-makers could be created, engendering even loftier dividend payouts and share appreciation for the companies' investors. That there were additional and plausible explanations for the narrowing difference in rates of infection between vaccinated and unvaccinated groups, that didn't indicate the need for booster shots, was ignored.

The need to rush shots into people's arms not only compromised safety but dictated dosing intervals as well. Every multiple-dose vaccine has a longer interval between the first and second dose than Covid-19 vaccines. For the shingles vaccine, the interval is two to six months. It's six months for the hepatitis A vaccine, one to two months for the hepatitis B vaccine, and a month to a year for the HPV vaccine. Yet the dosing interval for mRNA vaccines is only three to four weeks. That has puzzled vaccine experts. Why did Covid-19 vaccine manufacturers choose an anomalously short dosing interval?[25] According to the journal *Science*, some experts "have suggested that current Covid-19 dose spacing … was chosen not to provide long-lasting immunity, but to speed clinical testing."[26] Had a dosing interval of say, six months, been chosen, in line with the norm for multi-dose vaccines, drug manufacturers would have had to have waited many months to seek emergency use authorization. This would have necessitated a delay in the roll-out of vaccines to combat the United States' self-induced medical emergency, a gambit that would have been unacceptable to decision-makers. As a consequence, political, rather than pharmacological considerations shaped the dosing strategy, buttressed by the vaccine manufacturers' profit-making interests. Because the dosing interval was anomalously short, drug companies were able to seek authorization for emergency use much faster, and to start accumulating profits much sooner.

Scoop Sanger anticipated that cutting corners, "could create an opening for anti-vaccine activists to claim that [a vaccine] is untested and dangerous, and to spin reasonable concerns about the vaccine into widespread, unfounded fears about its safety."[27] It's unclear, however, why the ruling class journalist thought that what he called "reasonable concerns" about vaccine safety, based on inadequate testing, could, at the same time, be considered "unfounded fears." Surely, whatever trepidation people felt was not only justified but rational. At any rate, Sanger indirectly pointed out yet another reason why anyone contemplating a vaccine-centric strategy in the first half of 2020 was inviting failure: vaccine hesitancy. The phenomenon, at the best of times, would likely interfere with the project of achieving community protection, but by cutting corners in clinical trials, governments were exacerbating it.

In August of 2020, over one-third of US American adults said they were unlikely to take a Covid-19 vaccine. One in five said they were unlikely to accept inoculation, even if the pharmaceutical industry and government claimed it was safe and effective. Four months later, the numbers were unchanged.[28] A number of studies showed that people who refused to receive the vaccine were either concerned about vaccine safety, or believed the threat of Covid-19 to themselves was not great enough to warrant their accepting vaccine safety risks and side effects. While these views were regarded by many as deplorable, they were hardly irrational.

Many healthcare workers also refused to be vaccinated. Those who did cited a range of reasons for their refusal, including beliefs that:

- The vaccines were developed hastily.
- Vaccine policy was unduly influenced by pharmaceutical companies.
- Post-vaccination health problems were not being diligently reported and tracked.

They also pointed out the long-term effects of Covid-19 vaccines were unknown.[29]

As we have seen, the development of vaccines *was* rushed, and their rapid development was made possible only because a shortcut was taken on safety. The shortcut came in the form of emergency use authorization after only two months of a planned two years of safety and efficacy testing. As a consequence, billions of people were exposed to vaccines with no known long-term safety profile. Additionally, as we'll see, vaccine policy, as it related to boosters, was consistent with the preferences of the pharmaceutical companies, but contrary to the recommendations of the independent scientific advisory groups that counseled regulators. This accords with the judgment of vaccine-skeptical healthcare workers that vaccine policy was driven by the pharmaceutical industry, and that the policy was guided by profit motives without regard to safety. Finally, the view that post-vaccination health problems were not being diligently tracked and reported was not implausible. Having invested heavily in vaccines as the solution to the pandemic, and having inoculated millions of their own citizens, governments would not be inclined—indeed, they would be highly disinclined—to diligently gather data that could possibly show they had exposed their citizens unnecessarily to harm. The view of vaccine refusers, then, far from being unreasonable, uninformed, and unsophisticated, was the very opposite.

***

Vaccines and other drugs should not be used if there are safe alternatives that are equally or more effective, or if the potential dangers of the drugs or vaccines are greater than the risks of the disease they're intended to address. All drugs, including vaccines, are potentially harmful. Sometimes seriously adverse effects are deliberately hidden or overlooked by drug companies keen on making a profit. What's more, rare but severe adverse reactions can evade detection in clinical trials and only become evident after a drug has been given to millions of people.

In November 2000, David Healy, an Irish psychiatrist, was offered a position as clinical director at the University of Toronto's Centre for Addiction and Mental Health. He was invited to the university to give a talk on the limitations of clinical trials in medical research. Healy dwelled on a known problem: Adverse side-effects that are too rare to be observed in a clinical trial. Healy drew attention to Prozac, a drug that Harvard psychiatrist, Martin Teicher, had argued increased the probability of suicide in its users. While Prozac's manufacturer had claimed the drug had been found to be safe in clinical trials, the Irish psychiatrist agreed with Teicher that Prozac increases the chances users would take their own lives. Unfortunately for Healy, Prozac's manufacturer, Eli Lilly, provided over 50 percent of funding for the clinic Healy was to lead. Soon after his talk, the university withdrew Teicher's job offer. It was later discovered that the drug company had covered up evidence from its clinical trials of some adverse reactions to Prozac. GlaxoSmithKline, the manufacturer of a similar drug, Paxil, had done the same with its clinical trials.[30]

The Healy episode revealed two important facts relevant to vaccination. First, rare adverse side effects may not show up in trials. This danger would seem to be especially acute if trials are fast-tracked and drugs are approved for emergency use. Second, profit-seeking can lead pharmaceutical companies to cover up negative clinical trial data.

In the 1990s, Nancy Olivieri, a hematologist and director of the University of Toronto's Hospital for Sick Children Program of Hemoglobinopathies, was involved in a trial of deferiprone, a drug used in the treatment of the blood disease, thalassemia major. The drug was manufactured by Apotex, which, at the time, was in negotiations with the university to make a major donation. During the course of the trial, Olivieri discovered that the drug was potentially lethal. Apotex threatened to take legal action if she disclosed her findings publicly. Undeterred, Olivieri published her research in the *New England Journal of Medicine*, triggering her dismissal. She was later reinstated.[31] Significantly, Apotex sought to cover up the grave potential harm of its drug.

Merck, the drug company that received subsidies from the US government to help Johnson & Johnson manufacture its Covid-19 vaccine and to develop the antiviral pill, Molnupiravir, pleaded guilty to criminal charges after it was found to have manipulated trial data for the painkiller, Vioxx. Vioxx was implicated in heart failure in tens of thousands of users.[32] Other companies have also misrepresented safety and efficacy data.

According to *The Intercept*, "Pfizer paid $2.3 billion in criminal and civil fines to settle allegations that the company illegally marketed several drugs for off-label purposes that were specifically not approved by the Food and Drug Administration. The company instructed its marketing team to advertise Bextra, which was approved only for arthritis and menstrual cramps, for acute and surgical pain issues." Off-label use of Bextra placed patients at risk of heart attack and stroke. John Kopchinski, an employee who blew the whistle on Pfizer, revealed that the company's commitment to sales (i.e., profits) was so strong, it encouraged employees "to sell drugs illegally," even if it meant endangering the health of users.[33] Pfizer, of course, is the manufacturer, with BioNTech, of the world's top selling Covid-19 vaccine.

To deter drug companies from putting their quest for profit ahead of protecting the public from harm, governments mete out heavy fines to firms that are caught covering up the hazards of their products. But the drug companies build reserves into their budgets to cover the cost of the fines. The reserves are made possible by the drug companies' practices of charging their customers exorbitant fees and paying their employees less than the value of their labor.[34] In the end, government fines aren't much of a deterrent, if the potential profits of selling an unsafe drug exceed the cost of the fine, and drug companies accept fines as the cost of doing business.

In their book *The Illusion of Evidence-Based Medicine*, pediatric psychiatrist Jon Jureidini and philosopher Leemon McHenry argue that profit-making corrupts the clinical trials used to assess the safety and efficacy of drugs.[35] Because the development of drugs is expensive, drug makers stand to lose money if new drugs don't pan out. What's more, if clinical trials reveal drugs to be unsafe or ineffective, the drug makers are denied access to rich veins of future profit. Drug manufacturers, then, have an enormous incentive to manipulate and interpret clinical trial data to make unsafe drugs appear to be safe, and ineffective drugs appear to be effective. This can include running trials multiple times until, by chance, positive results are produced, hiding data, cherry-picking data, or outright misrepresentation of results.

Many people at the very least intuit that drug companies, as entities driven by profit, are untrustworthy. Many consumers distrust Big Pharma's pronouncements on the safety and efficacy of its products, for good reason. The pharmaceutical industry is not exempt from the warning *caveat emptor* (buyer beware). And because every time a consumer uses one of Big Pharma's products they accept a risk to their health, it's all the more important to pay heed to the warning when buying drug company products. This is not to say that Covid-19 vaccines are unsafe and ineffective. To be sure, capitalist incentives motivate drug companies to introduce unsafe and ineffective drugs if they can get away with it, but it doesn't follow that all drugs developed by Big Pharma are ineffective and potentially harmful. It's just that it's hard to know. What's more, with ruling class politicians in Washington appointing Big Pharma insiders to lead the FDA—and worse, industry insiders who believe the regulatory burden on drug companies is too great—the warning, buyer beware, is as important as ever, if not more so. When people have cogent reasons to doubt the safety and efficacy of the drugs capitalist pharmacy develops, and which industry-insider regulators authorize, they adopt a precautionary attitude. And precautionary attitudes are all the stronger when the disease a vaccine is used to prevent is seen as a minor risk.

***

The direct risk of Covid-19 to individuals is small. The vast majority of people infected by SARS-CoV-2 survive. Even for the majority of people 65 years and older, the novel coronavirus is not a death sentence. And most people who are sickened by Covid-19 experience only mild to moderate symptoms. Some even experience no symptoms, unaware they have the disease. It's true that Covid-19 has hospitalized many people and caused millions of premature deaths. But the number of people the contagion has hospitalized and killed pales in comparison with the number of people who were infected but weren't hospitalized and didn't die.

This doesn't mean, however, that Covid-19 isn't a danger. It is. While not a significant individual risk (unless you are elderly, immunosuppressed, or have an underlying condition), it is a grave societal danger. Unless measures are taken to curb its spread, the virus will make enough people severely ill all at once that hospital capacity will be exceeded and medical resources overwhelmed. If medical systems crash, the societal dangers escalate. Surgeries are cancelled. People requiring urgent care for other conditions are turned away from hospitals. People don't show up for work because they're frightened or need to stay at home to care for loved ones who are ill, or are ill themselves. Economies are plunged into chaos. In proportion as the virus rips through the population, the societal crisis grows.

Viewed from the perspective of an individual—especially one who is young and healthy—Covid-19's health risks are vanishingly small. The merits of vaccination for the individual, depend on two questions: What are the chances of permanent injury or death by the disease? For Covid-19, low. What are the chances of permanent injury or death by the vaccine? For Covid-19 vaccines, also low, as far as we know, for most people. However, Covid-19 vaccine risks to personal health, while low, may still be higher than the risks of the disease, depending on who you are. And there is reasonable room for doubt about the safety of Covid-19 immunizations. They may be less safe than acknowledged, for the reasons cited above.

I point this out, not to support the anti-vax position—which I reject, for reasons to be explained in a moment—but to show that from the perspective of the individual, and especially from the point of view of young and healthy individuals, the refusal to accept Covid-19 vaccination is far from an irrational and indefensible position. Because there are valid reasons to question the safety of Covid-19 vaccines, there are reasonable grounds to expect Covid-19 vaccine hesitancy to flourish. A vaccine strategy that fails to take vaccine hesitancy into account, and does nothing to extirpate its underlying causes, is flawed. Or, to put it another way, if you want people to accept vaccination, don't lie to them that the pharmaceutical industry sets public health as its highest priority (when it sets profits as its only priority); don't mislead them that "industry-captured" regulators work to protect the public (when they work to protect the interests of industry shareholders); and don't tell them that capitalist pharmacy works for them (when it works for capitalists first and the public only incidentally, if at all). Deception breeds mistrust. The way to allay vaccine hesitancy is to take profit-seeking out of the pharmaceutical industry—to reconstitute the industry on a non-profit basis, making its enterprises answerable to democratic bodies, rather than to the imperative of profits and profit-seeking investors.

While a reasonable individual might decide that the health risk of a Covid-19 vaccine is greater than the personal risk of the disease itself—especially in light of the multiple reasons to exercise caution in accepting assurances that vaccine-risk is low—there are strong societal reasons for accepting vaccination, if vaccination is the only feasible way within current constraints to safeguard healthcare systems and to avoid the multiple crises that would ensue were hospitals overwhelmed and medical resources overstressed.

The best societal approach to the problem of Covid-19 is a zero-Covid strategy, and ultimate exit from the pandemic through community protection achieved by mass inoculation, employing vaccines that have been assessed to be safe and effective in full clinical trials carried out over a period of more than one year, and produced by public sector enterprises regulated by bodies that are directly answerable to the public. However, with capitalism ascendant, the best societal approach has not been on the agenda in large parts of the world. What, then, is the best approach, given that the dominant strategy in most "capitalist-captured" countries is flattening the curve? Flattening the curve means herd immunity achieved over a prolonged period during which public health restrictions are alternately imposed and lifted to protect hospitals. Under this scenario, most people eventually fall ill from Covid-19, and many millions die. The pandemic ends when most people acquire immunity through infection.

In contrast, mass uptake of vaccines offers an alternative route out of the pandemic through vaccine-acquired community protection (herd immunity achieved through vaccination). This has the advantage of achieving community protection quickly and obviating the need to produce herd immunity through natural infection. Natural infection-acquired herd immunity is a slow process, requiring ongoing public health restrictions to protect hospitals from undue strain. Ultimately, it engenders a mountain of corpses. Community protection achieved through vaccination means a faster exit from the pandemic and fewer deaths.

Unfortunately, owing to vaccine refusal, the vaccine-centric approach metamorphosed into a hybrid model for exiting the pandemic. Population immunity would be achieved through both vaccination (quickly) and, for the unvaccinated, infection (drawn out over a prolonged period in which public health emergency measures would need to remain in effect). The irony was that the people who refused to be vaccinated were often the same people who objected to public health restrictions, yet their refusal to accept vaccination guaranteed the restrictions would carry on.

***

A puzzle. In 2020, the Rockefeller Foundation presented a proposal to the Trump administration to tackle the Covid-19 pandemic. Invest $100 billion in a health corps of 300,000 public servants to conduct a country-wide test, trace, and quarantine program, emulating the strategy that allowed China to bring its outbreak under control and safely reopen its economy.[36] The White House declined. Instead, Washington decided to spend tens of billions of dollars on a vaccine program, supported by the logistical expertise of the US military. That same military logistical capability could have been leveraged to create and operate a test, trace, and isolate program. It wasn't. Why, with the pandemic upon it, would Washington turn down an approach to pandemic control that had been shown to be successful in China, in favor of going all in on a vaccine program which, in the first half of 2020, appeared to any reasonable person to have little chance of success? Why pass on the sure thing and bet on the long shot?

The decision seems irrational. In the early days of the pandemic, no one knew whether humans could produce immunity to SARS-Cov-2. If not, a vaccine was out of the question. If so, there was less than a 10 percent chance, based on the history of vaccine research, that a shot could be found to do the job. And since the shortest time ever to develop a safe and effective vaccine was four years, by the time a vaccine arrived, it might be too late. Moreover, the experience of other politicians who had promised a vaccine as the solution to an epidemic should have been sobering. In 1981, Richard Schweiker, Ronald Reagan's secretary of health, promised an AIDS vaccine in two years. In 1991, Bill Clinton boldly declared that an AIDS vaccine would be developed before the decade was out. "It is no longer a question of *whether* we can develop an AIDS vaccine," the president said. "It is simply a question of *when*."[37] These failed auguries surely should have provided occasion for pause. Meanwhile, China had cracked the code. By implementing stringent public health measures, the giant East Asian country had effectively beaten Covid-19 and reopened its economy. Here was a model for how to deal effectively with the pandemic, and yet Washington chose to roll the dice on vaccines. Why?

Another puzzle. Washington said time was of the essence, and that a vaccine needed to be rolled out quickly. Why, then, bet on untried technologies, when older, established, inactivated and attenuated virus technologies could be quickly pressed into service? Proponents of the new technologies said they allowed vaccines to be developed faster than would be true of older technology. But the Chinese pharmaceutical firm, Sinopharm, used the so-called older, slower way of developing a vaccine, and produced its shot as quickly as Pfizer, Moderna, and AstraZeneca did theirs.

Still another puzzle. Messenger RNA vaccines presented multiple logistical difficulties. The vaccines needed to be stored at extremely low temperatures, requiring special refrigeration equipment. This made distribution difficult and expensive, especially in low- and middle-income countries. Older, proven, technology, in contrast, could be distributed more easily, and at far lower cost. Why then choose a vaccine that would be difficult to distribute, when time was of the essence?

All down the line, Washington made choices that appeared to have the least chance of success. It chose vaccination, when the *a priori* probability of success was under 10 percent, instead of selecting elimination, which China and a few other countries had showed worked remarkably well. It chose completely novel vaccine technologies, with no track record, over established technologies with undoubted success for a number of diseases. And it invested in mRNA vaccines, which would be expensive and difficult to distribute, and impractical for use in poor countries, over vaccines that could be more easily distributed.

Part of the puzzle can be explained by the financial interests of the people who chose the vaccine candidates in which Operation Warp Speed would invest. Moncef Slaoui had a substantial owner-ship stake in Moderna. When he and his team chose Moderna to receive over $2 billion in US government support, the com-pany's share price soared, bolstering Slaoui's already substantial wealth. William Erhardt and Rachel Harrigan, the Pfizer executives brought in to assist Slaoui in distributing taxpayer funding to US drug companies, benefited from the team's decision to select Pfizer as the second company to fill Operation War Speed's mRNA slot. But this explains little. The Slaoui team would not have been able to make self-aggrandizing decisions had a commitment not already been made to address the pandemic through vaccines. For Slaoui and his team to benefit from their Operation Warp Speed decisions, the program had first to exist. What made Washington commit to a vaccine program in the first place?

Part of the reason Washington favored the use of vaccines as the principal response to potential pandemic pathogens was the spade work Bill Gates had done in promoting vaccines as a world public health panacea. But it went deeper than that. Washington had long been planning for how to meet the threat of a biological attack, or warfare carried out with germs. Always, the response had been seen to depend mainly on developing and stockpiling two things: vaccines and personal protective equipment, or PPE.

Vaccines and PPE are not the only ways to address germ threats, but the idea is so ingrained in public discourse, that when asked how humanity ought to prepare for another pandemic, the answer is almost invariably: make sure we have enough respirators stock-piled and build vaccine manufacturing infrastructure. But there is another model of pandemic preparation that is almost always overlooked: develop the infrastructure to trace, test, and isolate. Few people—and no one in senior positions in government—ever talk about developing the infrastructure for an elimination strategy as the means to meet the next pandemic threat. Instead, the chorus only ever has two notes: vaccines and PPE.

This might reflect borrowed thinking from the military. The standard ways of defending military forces from weaponized pathogens are to equip troops with biohazard suits and respirators and to vaccinate them in advance against the bacteria, viruses, and other pathogens the enemy might employ. Test, trace, and isolate is absent from the military doctrine on defense against biological threats because it is ill-suited to the military environment. Blindly importing military anti-biological threat doctrine into public health practice omits an effective technique that, while ill-suited for military purposes, works very well for civilian ones.

Moreover, vaccines and PPE comport with the United States' techno-fix culture. "Techno-fixes," according to the late Howard P. Segal—who was an historian of science and technology at the University of Maine—"are short-term, avowedly practical proposed solutions to hitherto unsolvable economic and social problems" that "reflect an almost blind faith in the power of technology as panacea." Techno-fix culture biases people enmeshed in its web to overlook social and economic solutions, in favor of quick technological fixes. Segal pointed to a "continuing belief in techno-fixes amid the, at best, partial success of some and the utter failure of others."[38] Techno-fix culture, then, is a form of religion. Its votaries have faith that the god of technology will save humanity from all problems, despite the evidence. If techno-fix religion has a pope, it is surely Bill Gates.

But the techno-fix religion has other grand figures, as well. "Google," wrote historian Jill Lepore, "opened an R&D division called X, whose aim is 'to solve some of the world's hardest problems.'" Elon Musk, one of the world's richest people, if not, the wealthiest, promotes "a capitalism in which companies worry ... about all manner of world-ending disasters"—disasters, notes Lepore "from which only techno-billionaires, apparently, can save us."[39] The resonance with Gates' thinking is obvious.

US faith in technical prowess often leads the country astray, and to failure. Washington invested astronomical sums in building an Afghan military that was superior to the Taliban in numbers, training, equipment, and air power. The Afghan armed forces had 300,000 troops, an air force, and modern equipment, while the Taliban had only 75,000 fighters, inferior equipment, and no air force. Despite the Afghan military's US-supplied technical prowess, it was no match for a lightly armed band of peasants. In Korea, Vietnam, and Afghanistan, US technical prowess was defeated by peasant armies, just as in the war against Covid-19, US technical prowess was beaten by Chinese public health measures.

Explaining Washington's emphasis on pharmaceutical interventions at the expense of non-pharmaceutical ones as an outcome of the United States' religious faith in techno-fixes is helpful, but it doesn't explain where techno-fix culture came from. The almost blind faith in the power of technology as a panacea didn't emerge from a vacuum.

Bill Gates and other techno-billionaires promote techno-fix faith because the religion stimulates interest in their products. Techno-fix enterprises are the perfect distillation of Gates' view that the combination of technology and private enterprise can save the world. Technology and free enterprise are also the foundations of Gates', Musk's, and Bezos' fortunes and instruments of their fortunes' continued expansion.

The pharmaceutical industry is the perfect techno-fix industry. Is your blood pressure too high? Why lose weight, join a gym, and reduce salt intake, when you can take a diuretic? Suffering from gastroesophageal reflux disease (too much stomach acid)? You could stop drinking gallons of Starbucks every day, but why do that, when you can take a proton pump inhibitor? Is cholesterol gumming up your coronary arteries? Changing your diet will help, but a statin (cholesterol lowering drug) is the perfect techno-fix—an avowedly practical solution to an important problem. Pharmaceutical techno-fixes make drug companies and their investors rich. Exercise, weight loss, and diet modification don't. In fact, there's not much money to be made in promoting simple, effective measures to protect and improve public health. This is the most basic explanation for why Washington—dominated by investors—rejected the non-pharmaceutical public health measures that China and other countries had shown were capable of successfully containing the virus and shutting down community transmission. It's also the most basic explanation for why Washington pursued a private-sector-based vaccine techno-solution.

There were a number of other mutually reinforcing drivers of Washington's decision to define vaccination as "the key to getting the pandemic under control and keeping the economy strong,"[40] as Joe Biden put it, and which, at the same time, prompted Washington to reject a country-wide, fully-funded test, trace, and isolate program.

First, non-pharmaceutical public health measures are contra-indicated under capitalism. Rather than spending billions of dollars on vaccines, billions could have been spent on a robust public health response, of the type outlined by the Rockefeller Foundation and proposed to the Trump administration, shown to be effective by China, and recommended by the World Health Organization. But a public sector program to hire 300,000 public servants to conduct a country-wide test, trace, and quarantine program, to build quarantine facilities, to provide food, shelter and care to quarantined people, and then to pay the wages of the ill who were quarantined and unable to work, would offer few, if any, profit-making opportunities for the private sector. Shoe leather epidemiology—the basic, hard labor of tracking down infected individuals, tracing their contacts, and herding them into quarantine—is the unsung labor of public servants. On the other hand, vaccine production can be quickly and easily made a private sector activity.

Trump was so agitated by the thought that implementing public health measures would harm the production of profits, that he minimized the threat of the burgeoning outbreak to excuse his nonfeasance. "Trump grew concerned that any [strong] action by his administration would hurt the economy, and … told advisers that he [did] not want the administration to do or say anything that would … spook the markets,"[41] reported *The Washington Post*. Trump continued to downplay the Covid-19 calamity, even after he tested positive for the disease and was admitted to Walter Reed Medical Center. From his hospital room he encouraged people to be brave. "Feeling really good! Don't be afraid of Covid. Don't let it dominate your life," he tweeted. The ailing president trumpeted the great strides his administration was making in overseeing the production of US techno-fixes. "We have developed, under the Trump Administration, some really great drugs & knowledge."

Trump's approach was a capitalist *primum non nocere*, first do no harm, the physicians' code of avoiding interventions that harm the patient. Except, in Trump's case, the patient was big business. Whatever Trump did, his first rule was, don't hurt the big guys. US Americans could die by the bucketful, but Corporate USA and the stock market could not be harmed.

The Covid-19 denier in chief "cited his recovery from the contagion as evidence that businesses should fling open their doors because Covid 'is a treatable disease.'"[42] What he didn't mention was that the cocktail of monoclonal antibodies he received would very likely not be available to the average Covid patient turning up at a hospital gasping for breath. Position has its privileges, a reality Rudy Giuliani, Trump's lawyer and adviser, acknowledged after he too, stricken by the disease, received the same cocktail of drugs as Trump.[43]

Another driver of Washington's predilection for vaccines was the ability of billionaires, such as Bill Gates, to set the public health agenda to favor pharmaceutical solutions. Owing to their great wealth, billionaires, foundations supported by the wealthy and large corporations, and the pharmaceutical industry, were able to strongly influence public discourse on healthcare issues and to set the public policy agenda on matters related to health, including pandemic preparedness. They had long ago used their influence to push vaccines to the top of the agenda on how to meet the challenge of future pandemics. As a result, when the pandemic hit, governments followed the path capitalist influencers had already set.

Additionally, Washington—always a bastion of free enterprise and private sector boosterism—had no desire to promote the public sector as a solution to one of the twenty-first century's most important problems. The capitalist class, the US state, and individual billionaires such as Gates, agreed that capitalism is philanthropic and that free enterprise is the main vehicle through which the world's problems are to be addressed. There was no room in this view for the public sector, except as a host for private enterprise parasitism and source of the private sector's new products.

The Centers for Disease Control and Prevention were hamstrung because they were associated with public health, which, to free enterprisers, bore the faint fetor of socialism. Additionally, they were seen as anti-business, a legacy of their battles to protect consumers from the deleterious health effects of tobacco and industrial pollutants. The centers could hardly, then, be given a prominent role in the fight against the novel coronavirus. The battle was to be treated as a grand opportunity for the business community to enlarge its wealth, not as a grand opportunity for the public sector to take center stage.

Trump deputed his vice president Mike Pence to head the White House Coronavirus Task Force, a further blow to public health. Pence was an advocate of small government—for the people, not for corporations and billionaires. A religious fanatic, he was the US version of the Taliban mullah. As governor of Indiana, he slashed the state's public health budget.[44] The chances of Pence's marshalling public health resources to combat the pandemic were approximately zero.

Writer and journalist Nina Burleigh observed that the White House's focus was "on its conviction that private enterprise was the way out of the disaster."[45] Not only would vaccines be the exit from the calamity, but vaccines produced by the private sector (generously funded by the public sector) would be presented as the only possible escape.

Burleigh also argued that the Trump administration's incompetence, evidenced in its failure to prevent hundreds of thousands of US citizens from dying, was deliberate. The White House could have seized the levers of public power to bring the pandemic under

control, but chose not to in order to avoid giving hope to US citizens that government alone, unhinged from its service role to the
bourgeoisie, could be a force for good.[46]

***

Against all odds, a number of vaccines were successfully developed
that regulators declared to be "safe and effective," so far as safety
and efficacy could be determined by severely truncated phase 3
clinical trials. With vaccines in hand, the architects of the vaccine
policy set out to sell their techno-fix as the Covid-19 panacea, with
the help of various opinion makers who could be relied on to promote a capitalist point of view. Joe Biden said that that vaccines had
given us "the upper hand against this virus" and announced that
we "can live our lives, our kids can go back to school, our economy
is roaring back."[47] Monica de Bolle, a senior fellow at the Peterson
Institute for International Economics, averred that "You can't
have functioning economies without vaccines."[48] *The Wall Street
Journal* described vaccines "as the only way out of" the pandemic[49],
while Canada's *Globe and Mail* announced that "Vaccines are the
best weapon in the war on COVID-19"[50] and "the most important
tool for fighting the virus."[51] Jeremy Farrar, director of the drug
company-endowed Wellcome Trust, and a scientific adviser to the
British government, agreed. Vaccines have "always been the exit
strategy from this horrendous pandemic,"[52] he declared. Two officials of the American Civil Liberties Union, David Cole and Daniel
Mach, opined that there "is no equally effective alternative [to
vaccines] available to protect public health."[53] *The New York Times'*
Donald G. McNeil Jr. rhapsodized about US "pharmaceutical prowess" and predicted it would allow the country to "bring the virus to
heel."[54] Nepal's health secretary, Laxman Aryal, intoned that the
only way to control the rate of infection—yes, the *only* way—was
through vaccination.[55] Meanwhile, French president Emmanuel
Macron announced that vaccination was "the only path back to a
normal life."[56]

Pundits and world leaders who anointed vaccines as the *only* solution, the *only* way out of the pandemic, and the *only* effective alternative, had either not heard that China, New Zealand, and South Korea, along with Vietnam and North Korea, had taken the exit out of the pandemic months earlier, or were repeating by rote nonsense pumped out of the White House, the Gates Foundation, and the pharmaceutical industry. One drug company executive had the audacity to declare that Big Pharma had "led the world in responding to this pandemic"[57]—a shocking misrepresentation. If anyone deserved credit for leading the world in responding to the Covid-19 crisis, it was the Communist Party of China, which protected 1.4 billion Chinese citizens from the virus's ravages, while minimizing the damage to the country's economy. Since China's economy was significantly integrated into the larger world economy as the world's largest market and world's largest manufacturer, Beijing's measures to eliminate community transmission in order to resume economic activity had the effect of minimizing economic impacts abroad, and safeguarding the substantial investments that North American, Western European, and Japanese investors had made in China. In contrast, Big Pharma led the world in only one way: cashing in on the Covid-19 calamity, arranging for its lickspittles and class cohorts in government to pick the US taxpayers' pockets to create a techno-fix to swell the wealth of drug company shareholders.

Big Pharma and its enablers in Washington hobbled the world response to the pandemic rather than led it. In late 2020, the Nepalese government reduced spending on non-pharmaceutical public health measures in order to husband resources to pay for vaccines, which it believed—as Washington and Big Pharma had told it often enough—were the exit ramp from the pandemic. "We can't overspend now and be left with nothing," said Nepal's health secretary, Laxman Aryal.[58] The Nepalese government stopped paying for anti-pandemic public health measures and diverted expenditures to vaccines. When the health secretary announced the country's change in direction, approximately 14 Nepalese were dying from Covid-19 daily. Six months later, the daily number had risen to over 200, in excess of a fourteen-fold increase. Shifting from an elimination to a vaccine-centric strategy hadn't set the stage for an exit from the pandemic—it had made Nepal's public health emergency worse.

The Nepalese government's decision to transition from non-pharmaceutical to pharmaceutical action, revealed a trade-off. The trade-off confronted not only Nepal, but a number of other countries. Governments had finite resources, and were unable to spend without limit on all the various possible ways of addressing the pandemic. Choices needed to be made. And the choices seemed to reduce to two possibilities: (1) Investments in robust non-pharmaceutical interventions, based on mass testing, contact tracing, quarantine, and support for the quarantined; or (2) Investments in pharmaceutical interventions, based mainly on vaccines but supplemented by therapeutics. Some governments, like Canada, Israel, and the European Union, tilted their pandemic spending toward vaccines, paying top dollars for vaccine doses to vault to the front of the queue. This allowed them to inoculate their citizens quickly, with a view to rapidly lifting restrictions on business activities. Other governments, like New Zealand, Australia, Singapore, and South Korea, tilted their pandemic spending toward elimination. This allowed them to supress community transmission, but delayed their access to vaccines.

Keen to open their economies,[59] a number of countries and jurisdictions, including the United States, Britain, and the Canadian province of Alberta, used the roll-out of vaccines to proclaim a "freedom day," when all, or most, public health restrictions, including wearing masks indoors, would be lifted. What happened next was at odds with the promise that vaccination would rescue the world from the pandemic. Instead of diminishing, infections and deaths from Covid-19 soared. This hardly looked like an exit.

While many adults had been vaccinated, many had chosen not to be, and some, as we have seen, had made this decision for sound reasons. Additionally, vaccines had yet to be approved for children.

As a result, a substantial proportion of the population remained unprotected. The effect, then, of lifting all public health measures, was to fully expose the unvaccinated to the hazards of the virus, denying them any protection, except that of the vaccines they refused to accept. A phrase was coined to explain what was happening. The pandemic had become "a pandemic of the unvaccinated."

Depending on one's definition of an "exit" from the pandemic, the vaccination strategy had either failed miserably or had the potential to succeed admirably. If an exit meant the virus had been virtually driven from human populations, arising only now and then in local outbreaks that were quickly contained, the vaccine strategy had failed miserably—and would always fail miserably. The initial crop of vaccines, while offering a high degree of protection against severe disease and hospitalization, would still leave many people vulnerable to mild or moderate disease, and did not prevent transmission. Consequently, even if every person on the planet were vaccinated, the virus would continue to circulate, and continue to make many people ill, though the number of people requiring hospitalization would be low enough to be accommodated by current hospital capacity.

Alternatively, were an exit from the pandemic defined as a level of community protection high enough that all public health restrictions could be lifted without straining hospital and medical resources, a pharmaceutical strategy could succeed. Success would depend on whether the following, working in combination, produced a sufficiently high level of community protection against hospitalization: (1) vaccination; (2) access to therapeutics, such as the antiviral drugs, to prevent hospitalization; and (3) immunity through previous infection. However, these conditions were not being met. Between the number of people who could not be immunized or refused inoculations and had not acquired natural immunity, the number of infections was still high enough to strain hospital and medical resources. On top of this, antiviral pills were still not available. As a result, some public health measures would need to remain in place, despite the mass availability of vaccines.

Vaccination had the potential to bring an end to the pandemic, under the relaxed definition of exit, but its potential had not yet been realized.

The response, apart from reintroducing some public health restrictions to relieve the strain on hospitals, was two-fold: The business community, and its allies in government, began to promote a strategy of "living with Covid," pressuring governments that had pursued an elimination strategy to lift their restrictions, especially border controls, in order to reopen the global economy. The second response was to promote the use of booster shots.

One by one, the elimination strategy countries yielded to business pressure, until only two countries remained in the elimination camp: China and North Korea. Inasmuch as North Korea had been isolated from the world economy, the capitalist world was indifferent to whether Pyongyang kept its borders closed. But China was another matter. As the world's manufacturing center, the world's largest market, and the site of vast Western investments, China came under considerable pressure from businesses in the US empire to open its borders and learn to live with Covid.

North American, Western European, and Japanese corporations with profit-making interests in China complained that Beijing's elimination strategy was hurting their bottom lines. While a weeks-long quarantine for anyone entering China prevented the virus from slipping into the country and protected Chinese citizens, it also created difficulties for foreign investors and executives who were trying to do business in the country. Business executives complained that China's border controls made business travel all but impossible. This created difficulties in attracting and retaining talent in Hong Kong and cut executives off from their families. What's more, shipping was delayed, disrupting supply-chains, by the requirement that ships' crews anchoring at Chinese ports undergo testing for the virus. Additionally, border controls discouraged Chinese citizens from leaving the country for tourism, depriving a number of countries of lucrative Chinese tourist revenue.[60] The Wall Street Journal complained that China's pandemic control measures "left business owners scrambling to pacify clients over delayed deliveries and … companies apologizing to share-holders for expected losses."[61] While acknowledging the truth that China's elimination strategy had been remarkably successful and was strongly supported by China's 1.4 billion people, the ruling class media in the US orbit nevertheless depicted China as an oddity—the national equivalent of King Canute, resisting what was presented as the inevitability of living with Covid.

The other response, the promotion of booster shots, was pure sham, and, more than that, criminal. The pharmaceutical com-panies argued, on the basis of inadequate data, that immunity was waning and that boosters were necessary but, at best, the data they presented suggested only that the vaccines had become less effect-ive in preventing mild or moderate disease. Primary vaccination continued to provide a high level of protection against hospitaliz-ation and death. And, as noted previously, there was an alternative explanation for what seemed like waning protection, namely, that the vaccinated and unvaccinated were becoming alike, because the unvaccinated were acquiring immunity through infection. At the same time, it could also have been true that the vaccinated were taking fewer precautions than they once had, believing falsely that immunization had made them invulnerable to infection. Whatever the case, there was no dispute that the vaccines remained highly effective in keeping people alive and out of the hospital. Accordingly, boosters would do nothing to relieve strain on med-ical resources. But they would add to the growing mountain of vaccine-maker profits, which was why Pfizer-BioNTech, Moderna, and Johnson & Johnson promoted them.

Already, the companies' mRNA vaccines were the largest selling class of drug in history.[62] The Pfizer-BioNTech vaccine was Pfizer's best selling drug of all time, accounting for over half of its third quarter revenue in 2021.[63] The challenge for the two companies was how to keep the gravy train rolling. The obvious answer was to build a case that boosters were needed now and that regular boosting would be needed far into the future.[64] Pfizer announced that people would need to be vaccinated annually, if not every six months, though it had not a speck of evidence that this was true. Moderna's president Stephen Hoge declared—also, without a jot of evidence—that boosters would be needed "annually, probably seasonally."[65] Dr. Science, Anthony Fauci, agreed. "Sooner or later you will need a booster," he intoned.[66] The White House—Big Pharma's executive committee—fell into line. In June 2021, the president made arrangements to buy one billion booster doses.

From the point of view of public health, there were two compelling reasons why the White House booster decision was wrong. First, vaccines can be harmful, and therefore should not be administered unless the potential benefit outweighs the potential harm. Whenever vaccines are given to billions of people, thousands die, more are permanently injured, and many more are stricken by illness. To be sure, from the perspective of an individual, vaccine risks may be very low. But if the chance of dying from a vaccine is only one in one million, the vaccine will, despite this low individual risk, kill nearly 8,000 people, if administered universally. Regarding mRNA vaccines, young males have an elevated risk of developing myocarditis, but also a very low risk of hospitalization or death from Covid-19. The dangers of vaccination for this group preponderate the benefit. It is unethical to expose people to the potential harm of a vaccine if there is no evidence of benefit. In the case of boosters, there was no evidence that additional doses would produce advantages in reduced hospitalization and lower mortality. Drug company data showed that the vaccines were 90 percent effective against hospitalization.[67] "You want this vaccine to protect against the kind of illness to cause you to seek medical attention, or be hospitalized," remarked Paul A. Offit, a member of the Food and Drug Administration's vaccine advisory committee. "And until you see any evidence that that isn't true, then you don't need a booster dose."[68]

The second reason the Biden administration's booster decision was detrimental to public health was that administering unnecessary vaccine doses to people who were already protected from serious illness and hospitalization denied doses to people in poor countries whose governments lacked the means to compete with rich countries for the limited vaccine supply. The vaccine makers' refusal to share their recipes with manufacturers that had idle capacity, and could make generic copies, artificially restricted the global stockpile. Healthcare workers and vulnerable populations in poor countries were forced to wait for primary doses, while the rich countries paid top dollars for doses they didn't need and the vaccine manufacturers watched their mountains of profit grow ever higher. This was not only morally indefensible, since it created a vaccine apartheid, but was also scientifically bone-headed, since it slowed the world's exit from the pandemic by allocating vaccine resources to where they were needed least and away from where they were needed most. As WHO director-general Tedros said, "Blanket booster programs are likely to prolong the pandemic, rather than ending it, by diverting supply to countries that already have high levels of vaccination coverage, giving the virus more opportunity to spread and mutate."[69]

But while there were compelling public health reasons to forgo boosters, there were cogent profit-making reasons to promote them. From the point of view of capitalist pharmacy, boosters were desirable. They meant rich countries would continue to pay top dollars for limited doses. If this exposed people in high-income countries unnecessarily to vaccine health hazards (such as myocarditis in young males), and forced people in low-income countries to wait for primary doses, so be it. Profits mattered. Humanity didn't. In effect, the best the vaccine-makers could do was present evidence their vaccines may, yes, *may*, have become less protective against *mild to moderate* disease, but had no evidence their vaccines had become less effective against hospitalization and death. In other words, they had no evidence boosters were needed, but they did have an insatiable need for the profits which booster sales would provide. Monica Gandhi, a professor of medicine and infectious disease specialist at the University of California, San Francisco, worried that Washington's endorsement of boosters reflected "a profit motive ... rather than sound scientific reasoning."[70]

The White House's decision to echo Pfizer's and Moderna's call for boosters produced indignation at the FDA. The director of the agency's vaccine office, Dr. Marion Gruber, and her deputy, Dr. Philip Krause, announced they would retire early, in protest. The booster decision should have been taken by FDA career scientists, based on the evidence, the director and her deputy averred. By endorsing boosters before the FDA had determined whether they were safe, effective, or necessary, not only was the White House breaking a promise to "follow the science," it was pressuring the regulatory agency to kowtow to political demands (and while they didn't say so, behind those political demands lay the profit-making demands of Big Pharma). What's more, Gruber maintained there was no evidence that booster shots were needed.[71] Jason L. Schwartz, a professor of health policy at Yale University, pointed out that Biden had inverted the drug approval process: the White House should only have endorsed a vaccine after it had been evaluated and approved by the agency, not before.[72] Instead, the White House was endorsing boosters before government scientists had a chance to evaluate them. Biden expected the FDA and CDC to rubber stamp his decision, which, in turn, was a rubber stamp of Moderna's and Pfizer-BioNTech's plans. By November 2021, federal regulators had dropped the practice of consulting with independent panels of outside vaccine experts, after the panels recommended against the broad use of boosters, contrary to Biden's—and the vaccine-makers'—wishes.[73] Significantly, Biden's pressure on regulators to ignore the science was of a piece with the practice of the Trump administration. It had pressured regulators to approve hydroxychloroquine and convalescent plasma as treatments for Covid-19, absent any evidence they worked.

In the wake of Gruber's and Krause's announcement of early retirement, an international group of scientists published an article in *The Lancet* echoing the FDA scientists' view that there wasn't nearly enough evidence to justify additional vaccine doses. The scientists said that they had found that the vaccines were 95 percent effective against severe disease, and were more than 80 percent effective in protecting against infection. While they acknowledged that boosters might eventually be needed, they said that extra doses should only be used if there is clear evidence that the benefits outweigh the risks. That evidence, they pointed out, was missing. The scientists countered that more lives would be saved if vaccines were deployed to poor countries and urged rich countries to focus on this task.[74]

Despite the objections of scientists, the FDA and CDC approved Pfizer's booster application. The company's submission was based on a small study of 300 subjects showing that booster shots produced an increase in neutralizing antibodies. This finding was beside the point. While it indicated that an extra dose could boost immunity, it didn't show that immunity based on primary vaccination was inadequate and that a booster was therefore needed. Pfizer's presentation was akin to saying that four meals a day increases one's sense of satiety, not that four meals a day is necessary. Moreover, boosters are not required for other vaccines that prevent severe disease or hospitalization. Authorizing the use of a Pfizer-BioNTech booster would treat the companies' inoculation as a special case, though it was not clear on what scientific or public health grounds a Covid-19 vaccine was to be treated as being unique.

There was, however, a political and economic basis for this decision. The Biden administration had no other measures to combat the continuing pandemic but vaccines, having ruled out elimination, and, by this point, even mitigation, in favor of living with Covid. Promoting boosters created the impression (a false one) that the administration was taking steps to rein in the virus while, at the same time, indulging Pfizer's and BioNTech's shareholders, always a top priority for the White House. A final point: the long term safety profile of Pfizer-BioNTech's primary vaccine had never been established. Phase 3 clinical trials, planned for two years, had been effectively terminated after only a few months. But at least these trials involved large numbers of participants. In its booster application, Pfizer-BioNTech relied on data from only 300 participants. The robustness of their data was limited, both in the number of subjects, and the length of time over which booster safety was assessed. In other words, if the vaccine-makers had limited data on the safety of their primary doses, they had even less data on the safety of their booster doses.

Soon after, the FDA also approved Moderna's and Johnson & Johnson's boosters, despite clear inadequacies in the companies' data supporting their applications. Moderna did not profess that a booster to prevent severe disease or hospitalization was needed, but asked for approval anyway, its appetite for a continuing stream of revenue motivating its application. Moreover, it was unable to meet all of the FDA's criteria for a booster shot. And frighteningly, the company failed to provide sufficient safety data. Despite these failures, Moderna's booster was approved. The regulators reasoned that if recipients of the Pfizer-BioNTech vaccine were authorized to receive a booster, then recipients of the Moderna vaccine would need to be granted the same privilege.[75] Already, Moderna's primary vaccine had been approved on the basis of limited safety data. Now, regulatory safeguards were being lifted altogether. Moderna was being granted approval to subject hundreds of millions of people to a booster on which there was not one jot of evidence the inoculation was safe. The FDA and CDC, acting under pressure from the White House, had completely abandoned whatever integrity they had as guardians of public safety.

If authorization of the Moderna booster was a travesty and potentially injurious to the public, approval of an extra Johnson & Johnson dose was criminal. In its submission, the company produced data based on only 17 volunteers—far too few to arrive at any meaningful conclusions about either safety or efficacy. Worse, the company's data were not verified by the FDA.[76] Regulators said that since they approved additional Pfizer-BioNTech and Moderna doses, they would have to approve additional Johnson & Johnson doses.[77] In making this decision, the FDA repudiated its role as tribune of public health, jeopardizing the safety of millions in order to allow Johnson & Johnson to share in the booster bonanza.

Despite the Biden administration's success in approving boosters on the drug manufacturers' behalf, vaccine experts, the WHO director-general, and WHO scientists continued to speak out against unnecessary doses. They argued that primary vaccination continued to provide protection against hospitalization and death; that the pandemic continued to be fueled by those who had not received primary immunization; and that all efforts should be directed at vaccinating the unvaccinated. They might have added that neither Pfizer-BioNTech, Moderna, or Johnson & Johnson showed that boosters were necessary, and that the companies were unable to present data that their boosters were safe. While these arguments may have slowed uptake of extra doses, the emergence of the Omicron variant, and the panic that ensued, provoked high-income countries to step up their booster campaigns and their citizens to line up for third doses (and in Israel fourth doses), misled by their leaders that an extra dose was the best way to protect themselves from the new variant. In point of fact, there was no more evidence that boosters would provide enhanced protection against Omicron than there was that boosters would provide additional protection against any other variant. "The emergence of Omicron has prompted some countries to roll out booster programmes for their entire adult populations," noted the WHO director-general, "even while we lack evidence for the effectiveness of boosters against this variant."[78] He added, "We must be very clear that the vaccines we have remain effective against both the Delta and Omicron variants"[79] and that "No country can boost its way out of the pandemic."[80] Decisions were now being made by governments on how to combat the pandemic based on no science at all. However, the decisions buttressed Big Pharma's profit-making interests and were rooted in those interests. The decisions were also made despite the fact that all the tools for ending the pandemic were at hand, though the non-pharmaceutical tools continued to be shunned, now more than ever, as the White House insisted it was time to live with Covid.

The Wall Street Journal observed that "world leaders and chief executives" had decided their goal would be "to make life more normal" and to avoid a repeat of "2020 and 2021 when many businesses closed, offices were empty and schools went remote." Biden asked "Are we going back to March 2020?" His answer was: "Absolutely no!"[81] Thus, the White House—and most of the countries in the US orbit—would attempt to boost their way out of the pandemic—an impossible task, but one that was congenial to Big Pharma's top and bottom lines. Meanwhile, case counts in China—a country which had largely gone back to normal 18 months earlier—continued at their usual low level, free from an Omicron outbreak.

Recall that some healthcare workers refused to be vaccinated because they said vaccine policy was being driven by the pharmaceutical companies, motivated by profit-making goals, and indifferent to public safety. Clearly, they were not deluded. Vaccine policy was indeed being driven by the pharmaceutical companies, approved by industry-captured regulators, and promoted by a White House whose key members had ownership stakes in top vaccine makers. Eric Lander, the White House science adviser, owned up to $1 million in BioNTech shares. Susan Rice, Biden's domestic policy adviser, had a $5 million stake in Johnson & Johnson and owned up to $50,000 in Pfizer shares. Anita Dunn, who had been a senior Biden advisor, was managing partner at the consulting firm SKDK, a major Pfizer supplier.[82] The Latin phrase *salus populi suprema lex esto*, the health of the public is the highest law, was a manifest fiction. The reality was that in the United States and throughout the capitalist world, the highest law was the health of the investment portfolios of multimillionaires and billionaires.

CONCLUSION

The interests of capital and nothing but the interests of capital—here we have the guiding star towards which are directed all the activities of this robber band.
— N. Bukharin and E. Preobrazhensky[1]

The United States and China, the two largest countries in the world in GDP terms, pursued very different approaches to the Covid-19 pandemic. China acted quickly and decisively to expunge local outbreaks, while quarantining visitors for extended periods to block importation of the virus. This approach proved highly successful in safeguarding the health of Chinese citizens and minimizing the need for prolonged, universal, public health restrictions. True, China's restrictions were draconian by Western standards, but they were applied locally, and briefly. After two years of the pandemic, only 3.2 people per million had died of Covid-19, by far the lowest cumulative mortality rate of any major country. In contrast, over 2,479 US Americans per million were dead from the disease, many orders of magnitude greater.

Beijing's approach to the pandemic was also highly successfully in minimizing disruptions to the Chinese economy. Mass test, trace, and quarantine programs kept outbreaks to a minimum, allowing Chinese citizens to go about their daily lives with few restrictions. When lockdowns were imposed, they were brief and localized. As a result, China was able to reopen its economy quickly, and resume its economic growth, after only one quarter of recession. China's remarkable performance in protecting the health of its citizens, while at the same time minimizing the cost to its economy, is a significant public health achievement, and touchstone of how pandemics can be successfully managed, and, indeed, avoided altogether. Had the world emulated China's resolute public health choices in February and March 2020, when the Covid-19 threat was in its infancy, the pandemic would have been averted, and the lives of millions of people around the globe would have been spared. China demonstrated that pandemics are choices, not inevitabilities.

Rather than acting quickly to eliminate community transmission of SARS-Cov-2, the United States, and most other rich countries, tarried. Unwilling to impose measures that would disrupt business activity and interfere with the production of profits, they delayed. In the United States, the president, Donald Trump, refused to implement measures to prevent the spread of the virus, fearing that any action to combat the pathogen would acknowledge its existence and spook the markets. With the aim of safeguarding the investment portfolios of the wealthy, the denier-in-chief assured US citizens that all was well and that the virus would one day miraculously disappear. In contrast, China's leader, Xi Jinping, declared a "total war" on Covid-19. Not surprisingly, US denial led to US disaster. Few countries, large or small, saw as many people die per million from Covid-19 as did the United States. Most observers acknowledged that the US record in dealing with the pandemic was deplorable. Had Washington declared a total war, as Beijing had, it may have saved more than 800,000 US lives in the pandemic's first two years, the number of deaths that would have been prevented had the United States performed as well as China in controlling infection, adjusting for the size of the US population. The reality that many hundreds of thousands of US Americans died needlessly reveals that not only was the US record in responding to the pandemic disastrous, it was criminal. US decision-makers were aware of China's success and how it had been achieved. And yet they declined to emulate the successful Chinese model—based on old-school public health measures—and thereby condemned countless US citizens to death. Biden, whose pandemic performance was as execrable as Trump's, if not more so, is as much to blame.

While conceding that the US performance in protecting the health of its citizens was abysmal, most observers in the US orbit quickly added that the United States achieved one stellar success: the rapid development of vaccines. While it is debatable whether the United States developed vaccines any more rapidly than did Russia and China, even if we concede, *arguendo*, that US vaccines were the first to be developed—in the sense that they were approved for emergency use by the World Health Organization before any others—rapid vaccine development cannot be counted as a success, so much as an expedience. Covid-19 vaccines were only developed rapidly, and in record time, because the protocols that normally require multi-year evaluations of drug compounds for safety and efficacy were circumvented. Rather than carrying out human trials over many years, as is typical and necessary in routine vaccine development, drug companies, with government backing, fast-tracked the assessment of vaccine safety and efficacy. This was done because the United States and much of the rest of the world chose not to address their public health emergencies via the successful Chinese model, electing instead to implement hospital surveillance-based mitigation, while awaiting a vaccine—an approach they saw as comporting with their capitalist economies and supporting the interests of private investors. The head of the World Health Organization pointed out correctly on more than one occasion that all the tools to end the pandemic—including the non-pharmaceutical public health measures China had showed were effective in driving infections to near zero—were available; they merely had to be used. And yet, the tools, but for vaccines, remained idle and the pandemic continued. Having rejected the highly effective non-pharmaceutical interventions China had employed to great success, the United States had little else in its anti-Covid-19 arsenal but inoculations. For this reason, vaccine development was rushed, and vaccines were authorized for emergency use. One can hardly count as a significant achievement the unnecessary exposure of billions of people to vaccines whose safety had been inadequately assessed. The exposure was unnecessary because the emergency the vaccines was authorized to address was chosen, not inevitable. The proof of this was that in China, New Zealand, and South Korea, as well as Vietnam and North Korea, no public health emergency existed, at least until governments, China and North Korea excepted, caved to business pressure to "live with Covid."

***

The act of mobilizing public resources to achieve a public policy goal is not beyond the capabilities of the US government. And yet, if one believed the accounts of many observers, it is the absence of this capability that accounts for Washington's abysmally poor performance in responding to the pandemic. This explanation is nonsense. To develop, produce, and distribute Covid-19 vaccines the United States relied heavily on the public sector. The mRNA technology underlying Moderna's and Pfizer-BioNTech's vaccines was developed in publicly-funded university and government labs. BioNTech and Moderna licensed technology produced at the University of Pennsylvania, BioNTech additionally licensed a US government patent, and Moderna collaborated with the National Institutes of Health to produce what the NIH called the NIH-Moderna vaccine.[2] Washington shelled out billions of dollars in grants, subsidies, and advance purchase agreements to pharmaceutical companies to develop vaccines and therapeutics. Without public sector backing, Moderna, Pfizer, BioNTech, AstraZeneca, Johnson & Johnson and other pharmaceutical companies would never have taken on the task of developing and manufacturing Covid-19 vaccines and treatments; capitalist incentives would have discouraged it. Additionally, the logistical expertise of the Pentagon was pressed into service to ensure the vaccine makers got the materials they needed. The misnamed grand success of the

US Covid-19 response, namely, the rapid development of vaccines, would never have been possible had Washington not coordinated the entire affair centrally, drawing on public sector logistical and R&D support, and using its authority to tax the public and direct the resultant funds in desired ways. The public sector was a *sine qua non* of the vaccine response. Washington, then, is perfectly capable of mobilizing public resources to achieve public policy goals. Its efforts with vaccines demonstrate this to be so.

Washington could have used the public sector and its taxation authority to create a public health infrastructure to undertake mass testing, carry out contact tracing, and build quarantine facilities, as did China. Had Washington done this, community transmission of the virus would have been eliminated. Washington could have also quarantined travellers entering the country in government-run facilities, to prevent the importation of cases. Had Washington taken these steps, more than 800,000 US deaths would have been prevented in the first two years of the pandemic. If the Pentagon's resources and expertise had been mobilized to help make and distribute vaccines, they could also have been used to carry out mass testing, trace contacts, and build, staff, and maintain quarantine facilities in order to safeguard the health of US citizens. But this goal was never on Washington's agenda. Why not?

One reason is that tech super-billionaires—Bill Gates, Elon Musk, Jeff Bezos, and others—had promoted a techno-fix religion that defined private sector technology as the key to solving humanity's problems. They didn't invent the religion. It already existed. Nevertheless, as votaries themselves, with the means to promote their religion widely, they did much to strengthen the faith that humanity's most difficult problems would yield to profit-making technological solutions. What they concealed was that the private sector technology on which they had grown fabulously wealthy, and which they promoted as the solution to the world's ills, originated in public sector labs. The techno-fix religion demanded: (a) the continuing transfer of public sector technology to the private sector, (b) the use of public sector technology by the private sector to address grand problems, in order to (c) expand the tech billionaires' already vast wealth, and (d) present themselves, capitalist industry, and their class, as the keystone of human development.

The militarization of the United States also played a role in discouraging a public health response to the pandemic, and in focusing efforts on vaccine development. Capitalist imperatives have always driven the United States' economic elite—from plantation owners to manufacturers to financiers to tech lords—to reach beyond the territorial boundaries of the United States for profit-making opportunities. This led to the expansion of those boundaries, both formally, in the incorporation of territory, and informally, in the subsumption of foreign governments as vassals of a global US empire. "We believe," averred US vice president Kamala Harris, "that our growth should not stop at the water's edge."[3] And it hasn't. US capital has settled everywhere, nestled everywhere, and created connections everywhere. "More than 95 percent of the world's population lives beyond our borders," observed Biden, adding that "we want to tap those markets." Biden put the world on notice—as countless presidents have before him—that Washington will take "down trade barriers" that prevent US capital from tapping markets outside the United States.[4] How? The *ultima ratio regnum*, or the final argument of kings, of US economic expansion—the basis of US economic globalization—has always been military power. US military power opened markets abroad, keeps them open, and protects them from nationalists, socialists, communists, and foreign rivals. Today, as befits history's greatest empire, the United States is also history's greatest military colossus. Observers either celebrate or deplore the ability of the US investor class to project power globally, on terms unmatched by any other country at any other time, but none doubt it. The United States is the world's, and history's, most armipotent power, and its strong military orientation pervades its society. As a consequence, policy makers tend to think in military terms. A viral threat to civilian society is seen through the lens of the military, and the military offers a ready-made model for how to deal with it: vaccines and personal protection equipment. Hence, the military response to a bioweapons attack becomes the civilian response to a novel pathogen: inoculate the population and distribute masks.

Another reason why Washington favored vaccines over non-pharmaceutical public health measures was that an elimination strategy offered no profit-making opportunities for the private sector. There was no private sector infrastructure ready to carry out mass testing, to trace contacts, and to build, staff, and maintain quarantine facilities in early 2020, when the pandemic began. There was, however, a private sector pharmaceutical industry to which technology developed in publicly-funded labs could be transferred (and had long been transferred as a normal part of doing business), and which could then, with the ample assistance of the US state, be transformed into a Pantagruelian banquet of profits on which the capitalist class—including principals in the Trump and Biden administrations and the US Congress—could feast.

While it is conceivable that an elimination strategy could have been pursued in the United States based on private sector-provided testing, contact tracing, and quarantine-management, this was not a feasible option in 2020 and 2021. Instead, implementation of non-pharmaceutical public health measures would have had to have been a very large public sector affair. Mobilization of public sector resources for public benefit is inimical to a capitalist ideology that promotes the private sector as the most efficient and desirable way to address human needs. The last thing the wealthy elite in Congress, the administration, the media, the think tanks, and the country's boardrooms, wanted was a socialist solution to the pandemic, which is what a publicly-provided elimination project surely would have been. It would have been socialist in two ways: it would have been publicly-provided and planned; and the protection of public health—not the promotion of the profit-making interests of a wealthy few—would have been its aim.

Hence, under the sway of the capitalist class, Washington approached the viral crisis guided by a single question: How can this crisis be transformed into a money-making opportunity for an investor elite? The obvious answer, pre-conditioned by US faith in technological solutions, by US society's proclivity for solutions modelled on military responses, and by the unremitting quest for profits, was to exploit Covid-19 as a vast profit-making opportunity for Big Pharma.

To what public policy goal was the mobilization of vast public resources on behalf of Big Pharma directed? The goal was not to safeguard the health of the public. As much as it might be comforting to believe that the US government, and others in its orbit, acted with single-minded purpose to protect citizens from the dangers of SARS-CoV-2, the evidence indicates otherwise. These governments—dominated by the wealthy—acted to protect and promote the interests of the wealthy. They acted to provide the private sector—that is themselves and their class cohorts—the means to address the public health emergency of Covid-19 in a way that allowed them to expand their wealth. If the response created millions of preventable deaths; if it unnecessarily exposed billions to inadequately safety-tested vaccines, rushed into people's arms to address a preventable public health emergency; if it meant that vaccine technology was kept secret and not shared with humanity as a public good; all of this was of little consequence. For all that matters in a capitalist society are capitalists and their profits. Human lives are but the means to capitalist ends, to be sacrificed in vast numbers if necessary to the Moloch of profits.

Therein lies an important point. The goal of all public policy decisions in capitalist society is the promotion and protection of the profit-making interests of the society's eponymous class—capitalists. The interests of the public at large don't count, except so far as they contribute to the single, senior, over-arching goal of making the wealthy wealthier.

Could Washington have behaved differently? Might it have acted quickly and decisively in the early months of 2020 to destroy the infant pandemic in its womb? Could it have mobilized resources to undertake mass testing, contact tracing, and to build and operate quarantine facilities to eliminate community transmission of the disease and block its importation? Could it have used the public sector to manufacture and distribute vaccines, just as much as it used public resources to develop inoculations and help manufacture and distribute them? Might Washington have pursued a strategy of eliminating community transmission by non-pharmaceutical public health measures, while at the same time developing and testing vaccines at a pace adequate to assessing their safety and efficacy rather than rushing them into the arms of billions of people around the world before their safety had been fully evaluated? Could Washington have recognized that the common interests of humanity necessitated that all measures be taken to end the pandemic as quickly as possible and accordingly share vaccine technology, in order to expedite the delivery of vaccines to countries in the global south?

None of this was possible so long as public policy decisions were made by a capitalist state—that is, by an apparatus of government dominated by billionaires, enmeshed in an ideological network of media, think tanks, and universities controlled by billionaires, operating from within a framework of capitalist strictures that limit the range of possible policy responses. To pursue elimination to save lives, to avoid the rushed development of vaccines, to share vaccine technology with humanity as a public good—that is, for the capitalist state to have acted in the interests of the public *contra* the interests of the capitalists—it would have been necessary for the capitalist state to have abolished itself. The rule of the billionaires would have had to have been brought to an end, and replaced by the rule of the public, in its own interest. In other words, the battle for democracy against the reign of plutocracy would have had to have already been won. Plutocrats will never abolish their own rule.

As it scythed through the world—or rather, as it scythed through most of the world outside of China and a few other countries—Covid-19 left a mounting pile of corpses in its wake. At the close of 2021, the official Covid-19 death toll was over 5 million, but many observers believed the true toll to be much higher, possibly 19 million.[5] SARS-Cov-2 was a killer. But it was a killer with a helper. Its henchman was capitalism. Capitalism discouraged governments from acting quickly and decisively to abort a public health crisis in embryo for fear of spooking markets and disrupting business activity. Capitalism stayed the hand of those who sought to implement the non-pharmaceutical public health measures that China demonstrated could quash the virus and allow economies to reopen quickly. Capitalism pushed governments to accept vaccines produced by private enterprise as the only exit from the pandemic and to rush them into people's arms before they were adequately tested. Capitalism forced the public to accept the economic risks and costs of vaccine development, while privatizing the economic gains. And after defining vaccines as the pandemic's off-ramp, capitalism prevented vaccine technology from being shared with humanity as a public good, slowing vaccine deployment around the world, delaying the day the viral holocaust would be a brought to an end. The killer's henchman was capitalism. No effective response to future pandemics is possible until the henchman is dead.

BIBLIOGRAPHY

A.B. Abrams, *Power and Primacy: The History of Western Intervention in the Asia-Pacific*, Peter Lang, 2019.

A.B. Abrams, *Immovable Object: North Korea's 70 Years at War with American Power*, Clarity Press, 2020.

Roy M. Anderson and Robert M. May, *Infectious Diseases of Humans: Dynamics and Control*, Oxford University Press, 1992.

John M. Barry, *The Great Influenza: The Story of the Deadliest Pandemic in History*, Penguin Books, 2018.

John Brewer, *The Sinews of Power: War, Money, and the English State, 1688-1783*, Harvard University Press, 1988.

N. Bukharin and E. Preobrazhensky, *The ABC of Communism*, Penguin Books, 1970.

Nina Burleigh, *Virus: Vaccinations, the CDC, and the Hijacking of America's Response to the Pandemic*, Seven Stories Press, 2021.

G. William Domhoff, *Who Rules America? Power & Politics*, McGraw-Hill Higher Education, 2002.

Friedrich Engels, *The Condition of the Working Class in England*, Penguin, 1987.

Ben Goldacre, *Bad Pharma How Drug Companies Mislead Doctors and Harm Patients*, McClelland and Stewart, 2013.

Donald Gutstein, *Not a Conspiracy Theory: How Business Propaganda Hijacks Democracy*, Key Porter Books, 2009.

Richard Horton, *The Covid-19 Catastrophe: What's Gone Wrong and How to Stop it Happening Again*, Polity, 2020.

Jon Jureidini and Leemon B. McHenry, *The Illusion of Evidence-Based Medicine: Exposing the Crisis of Credibility in Clinical Research*, Wakefield Press, 2020.

Roger Keeran and Thomas Kenny, *Socialism Betrayed: Behind the Collapse of the Soviet Union*, International Publishers, 2004.

Michael Lewis, *The Premonition: A Pandemic Story*, W.W. Norton & Company, 2021.

Mariana Mazzucato, *The Entrepreneurial State: Debunking Public vs. Private Sector Myths*, Public Affairs, 2015.

Linsey McGoey, *No Such Thing as a Free Gift: The Gates Foundation and the Price of Philanthropy*, Verso, 2015.

Jacques R. Pauwels, *The Myth of the Good War: America in the Second World War*, James Lorimer and Company, 2002.

Robert A. Pape, *Dying to Win: The Structural Logic of Suicide Terrorism*, Random House, 2006.

Laurence H. Shoup, *Wall Street's Think Tank: The Council on Foreign Relations and the Empire of Neoliberal Geopolitics, 1976-2014*, Monthly Review Press, 2015.

Laurence H. Shoup and William Minter, *Imperial Brain Trust: The Council on Foreign Relations and United States Foreign Policy*, Authors Choice Press, 2004.

Frank W. Snowden, *Epidemics and Society: From the Black Death to the Present*, Yale University Press, 2020.

Roderick Stewart (Ed.), *The Mind of Norman Bethune*, Fitzhenry and Whiteside, 2002.

Albert Szymanski, *The Capitalist State and the Politics of Class*, Winthrop Publishers, Inc., 1978.

Albert J. Szymanski and Ted George Goertzel, *Sociology: Class, Consciousness, and Contradictions*, D. Van Nostrand Company, 1979.

David Vine, *The United States of War: A Global History of America's Endless Conflicts, from Columbus to the Islamic State*, University of California Press, 2021.

William Appleman Williams, *The Great Evasion*, Quadrangle Books, 1964.

William Appleman Williams, *The Tragedy of American Diplomacy*, W.W. Norton & Company, 2009.

NOTES

Preface

1. Friedrich Engels, in Lewis S. Feuer's Socialism: Utopian and Scientific, in (Ed.), *Marx & Engels: Basic Writings on Politics and Philosophy*, Doubleday, 1989, p. 99.
2. WHO Director-General's opening remarks at the WTO - WHO High Level Dialogue: Expanding COVID-19 Vaccine Manufacture to Promote Equitable Access, 21 July 2021.
3. WHO Director-General's opening remarks at the WTO - WHO High Level Dialogue: Expanding COVID-19 Vaccine Manufacture to Promote Equitable Access, 21 July 2021.
4. Carolyn Y. Johnson and Tyler Page, "Moderna plans to build vaccine plant in Africa to produce 500 million doses a year for lower-income nations," *The New York Times*, October 7, 2021; "One-off emergency tax on billionaires' pandemic windfalls could fund COVID-19 jabs for entire world," Oxfam.org, August 12, 2021.
5. Julia Musto, "Billionaire Bezos' Amazon warehouse employees depend on food stamps in 9 states," Fox Business, December 17, 2020.
6. Caitlin McCabe, "Companies Are Flush with Cash—and Ready to Pad Shareholder Pockets," *The Wall Street Journal*, May 16, 2021.
7. Ibid.
8. Peter Loftus, "Who invented Covid-19 vaccines? Drugmakers battle over patents," *The Wall Street Journal*, December 29, 2021.

1. The Killer

1. Holman W. Jenkins, Jr. "What India's Viral Misery Is Telling Us," *The Wall Street Journal*, April 30, 2021.
2. Hu Xijin, "History will remember China's achievements and US' shames in COVID-19 battle," *Global Times*, January 13, 2021.
3. "COVID-19: Make it the Last Pandemic, The Independent Panel for Pandemic Preparedness & Response," World Health Organization, May, 2021.
4. https://sites.google.com/site/andyatkeson/
5. Brendan Sen-Crowe et al., "A closer look into global hospital beds capacity and resource shortages during the Covid-19 pandemic," *Journal of Surgical Research*, April, 2021.
6. Michael Worobey, "Dissecting the early COVID-19 cases in Wuhan," *Science*, November 18, 2021.
7. Ed Yong, "The New Coronavirus Is a Truly Modern Epidemic," *The Atlantic*, February 3, 2020.
8. John Gittings, "Hiding in Plain Sight: Why We Missed the Threat of a New Pandemic— and Other Existential Risks," *The Asia-Pacific Journal*, Japan Focus, July 15, 2021.

9. Frank M. Snowden, *Epidemics and Society: From the Black Death to the Present*, Yale University Press, 2019, pp. 6-7.

10. Frank M. Snowden, *Epidemics and Society: From the Black Death to the Present*, Yale University Press, 2019, p. x.

11. Betsy McKay and Phred Dvorak, "A Deadly Coronavirus Was Inevitable. Why Was No One Ready?", *The Wall Street Journal*, August 13, 2020.

12. Ed Yong, "The New Coronavirus Is a Truly Modern Epidemic," The Atlantic, February 3, 2020: Betsy McKay and Phred Dvorak, "A Deadly Coronavirus Was Inevitable. Why Was No One Ready?," *The Wall Street Journal*, Aug. 13, 2020.

13. Eric Levitz, "Why Humanity Will Probably Botch the Next Pandemic, Too," *The New York Magazine*, April 30, 2020.

14. Roy M. Anderson and Robert M. May, Infectious Diseases of Humans, 1991, cited in Richard Horton, *The Covid-19 Catastrophe: What's Gone Wrong and How to Stop it Happening Again*, 2020, p. 41.

15. Gail Wilensky, "The Importance of Re-establishing a Pandemic Preparedness Office at the White House," *The Journal of the American Medical Association*, July 9, 2020.

16. Robinson Meyer and Alexis C. Madrigal, "The Plan That Could Give Us Our Lives Back," *The Atlantic*, August 14, 2020.

17. A World at Risk, WHO, September 2019.

18. Uri Friedman, "We Were Warned," *The Atlantic*, March 18, 2020.

19. Ibid.

20. Ibid.

21. Betsy McKay and Phred Dvorak, "A Deadly Coronavirus Was Inevitable. Why Was No One Ready?", *The Wall Street Journal*, August 13, 2020.

22. www.macrotrends.net/countries/wld/world/population-density

23. Steven Lee Myers, Keith Bradsher and Chris Buckley, As China Boomed, It Didn't Take Climate Change into Account. Now It Must," *The New York Times*, July 26, 2021.

24. Frank M. Snowden, *Epidemics and Society: From the Black Death to the Present*, Yale University Press, 2019, p. 90.

25. Friedrich Engels, *The Condition of the Working Class in England*, Penguin, 1987, p. 71.

26. Ibid., p. 71.

27. John Gittings, "Hiding in Plain Sight: Why We Missed the Threat of a New Pandemic—and Other Existential Risks": *The Asia-Pacific Journal*, Japan Focus, July 15, 2021.

28. Ed Yong, "The New Coronavirus Is a Truly Modern Epidemic," *The Atlantic*, February 3, 2020.

29. Lynn C. Klotz and Edward J. Sylvester, "The unacceptable risks of a man-made pandemic," *The Bulletin of the Atomic Scientists*, August 7, 2012.

30. Alexandra Peters, "The global proliferation of high-containment biological laboratories: understanding the phenomenon and its implications," January 2019", *Revue scientifique et technique* (International Office of Epizootics), 37(3): 857-883.

31. Alison Young and Jessica Blake, "Here Are Six Accidents UNC Researchers Had With Lab-Created Coronaviruses," *ProPublic*, August 17, 2020.

32. Steve Connor, "Did lab leak from a laboratory cause swine flu pandemic?", *The Independent*, June 30, 2009.

33. WHO Director-General's opening remarks at the Member State Information Session on Origins, 16 July 2021.

34. The Editorial Board, "How Fauci and Collins shut down Covid debate," *The Wall Street Journal*, December 21, 2021.

35. From Upton Sinclair's 1935 book *I, Candidate for Governor: And How I Got Licked*.

36. Nina Burleigh, *Vaccinations, the CDC, and the Hijacking of America's Response to the Pandemic*, Seven Stories Press, 2021, p. 141.

37. Sarah Boseley, "Physiotherapy doesn't work for back pain, study says," *The Guardian*, September 24, 2004.

38. Frank M. Snowden, *Epidemics and Society: From the Black Death to the Present*, Yale University Press, 2019, p. ix.

2. The Response

1. Benjamin Mueller, "Will shortened isolation periods spread the virus?", *The New York Times*, December 28, 2021.

2. Grant Robertson, "The world's 'lost month' in fight against COVID-19," *The Globe and Mail*, May 12, 2021.

3. WHO Press Conference on Covid-19, August 4, 2021.

4. Eric Lander, "As bad as covid-19 has been, a future pandemic could be even worse — unless we act now," *The Washington Post*, August 4, 2021.

5. "COVID-19: Make it the Last Pandemic, The Independent Panel for Pandemic Preparedness & Response," World Health Organization, May, 2021, COVID-19: Make it the Last Pandemic (theindependentpanel.org).

6. "5 key terms for parsing Kim Jong un's vision for N. Korea, in 2022," *The Hankyoreh*, January 3, 2021.

7. Michelle Ye Hee Lee, "What's happening inside North Korea? Since the pandemic, the window has slammed shut," *The Washington Post*, September 9, 2021.

8. Choe Sang-Hun, "North Korea Declares Emergency After Suspected Covid-19 Case," *The New York Times*, July 25, 2020.

9. Howard Waitzkin, "COVID-19 in the Two Koreas," *Monthly Review*, September, 2021.

10. Michael Lewis, *The Premonition: A Pandemic Story*, W.W. Norton & Company, 2021, p. 99.

11. Amber Phillips, "Was the stock market the object of Trump's 'don't create a panic' coronavirus approach?" *The Washington Post*, September 10, 2020.

12. Yasmeen Abutaleb and Josh Dawsey, "Trump's soft touch with China's Xi worries advisers who say more is needed to combat coronavirus outbreak," *The Washington Post*, February 16, 2020.

13. "What did leaders of US, Japan and China say about COVID-19?" *The Hankyoreh*, March 14, 2021.

14. The source for all confirmed case and death figures is Our World in Data.

15. Rebecca Tan and Alicia Chen, "China's delta outbreak tests limits of zero-tolerance covid approach," *The New York Times*, July 29, 2021.

16. Michael Lewis, *The Premonition: A Pandemic Story*, W.W. Norton & Company, 2021, p. 85.

17. Talha Burki, "China's successful control of COVID-19," *The Lancet Infectious Diseases*, October 8, 2020.

18. Ibid.

19. Ibid.

20. Ibid.

21. Paul Hannon, Gabriele Steinhauser and Sha Hua, "Delta Variant's Spread Hobbles Global Efforts to Lift Covid-19 Restrictions," *The Wall Street Journal*, July 1, 2021.

22. Talha Burki, "China's successful control of COVID-19," *The Lancet Infectious Diseases*, October 8, 2020.

23. Liza Lin and Stella Yifan Xie, "Economic Costs Accumulate as Countries Worried by Delta Variant Extend Border Closures," *The Wall Street Journal*, September 11, 2021.

24. Keith Bradsher, "China Returns to Its Strict Covid Limits to Fight a New Outbreak," *The New York Times*, June 9, 2021.

25. Sha Hua, "Delta Variant Arrives in Wuhan After More Than a Year With No Covid-19," *The Wall Street Journal*, August 3, 2021.

26. Liu Caiyu, "Why can China confine flare-ups to dozens cases?" *Global Times*, May 18, 2021.

27. "What can the world learn from China's response to covid-19?" *The British Medical Journal*, December 2, 2021.

28. Miquel Oliu-Barton, "SARS-CoV-2 elimination, not mitigation, creates best outcomes for health, the economy, and civil liberties," *The Lancet*, April 28, 2021.

29. Steven Lee Myers, Keith Bradsher, Sui-Lee Wee and Chris Buckley, "Power, Patriotism and 1.4 Billion People: How China Beat the Virus and Roared Back," *The New York Times*, February 5, 2021.

30. Ibid.

31. William Mauldin, "Biden Defends Democracy at Summits With European Allies, Seeing China as 'Stiff' Competition," *The Wall Street Journal*, February 19, 2021.

32. Li Yuan, "In a Topsy-Turvy Pandemic World, China Offers Its Version of Freedom," *The New York Times*, January 4, 2021.

33. Justin Giovannetti, "The end of elimination: The abandonment of New Zealand's COVID-Zero strategy leaves few people pleased," *The Globe and Mail*, October 7, 2021; "No retreat from elimination! The New Zealand and international working class must fight to stamp out COVID-19," *The World Socialist Web Site*, October 8, 2021.

34. "Return to normal to start around Nov. 9, KDCA head says," *The Hankyoreh*, October 8, 2021.

35. Michael Lewis, *The Premonition: A Pandemic Story*, W.W. Norton & Company, 2021, p. 9.

36. KHN's, "'What the Health?': What Would Dr. Fauci Do?," November 19, 2020.

37. WHO Director-General's opening remarks at the media briefing on Covid-19, 14 December 2021.

38. WHO Director-General's opening remarks at the WTO - WHO High Level Dialogue: Expanding COVID-19 Vaccine Manufacture To Promote Equitable Access, 21 July 2021

39. WHO COVID-19 Virtual Press conference 3 August 2020.

40. Sarah Bahr, "Fauci Says It Could Be a Year Before Theater Without Masks Feels Normal," *The New York Times*, September 11, 2020.

41. Drew Hinshaw and Daniel Michaels, "Pfizer-BioNTech Covid-19 Vaccine Is Cleared for Use by EU Drug Agency," *The Wall Street Journal*, December 21, 2020.

42. Sarah Bahr, "Fauci Says It Could Be a Year Before Theater Without Masks Feels Normal," *The New York Times*, September 11, 2020.

43. Benjamin Mueller, "How a Dangerous New Coronavirus Variant Thwarted Some Countries' Vaccine Hopes," *The New York Times*, February 8, 2021.

44. Niharika Mandhana and Rachel Pannett, "As Coronavirus Surges in U.S. and Europe, Other Countries See One Case as Too Many," *The Wall Street Journal*, November 3, 2020.

45. Jon Kamp, Robbie Whelan, and Anthony DeBarros, "US Covid-19 deaths in 2021 surpass 2020'," *The Wall Street Journal*, November 20, 2021; Michelle Ye Hee Lee and Min Joo Kim, "North Korea has yet to begin coronavirus vaccinations as delays hamper U.N.-backed rollout," *The Washington Post*, August 24, 2021.

46. Niharika Mandhana and Rachel Pannett, "As Coronavirus Surges in U.S. and Europe, Other Countries See One Case as Too Many," *The Wall Street Journal*, November 3, 2020.

47. Eric Reguly, "Why herd immunity to COVID-19 is proving elusive – even in highly vaccinated countries," *The Globe and Mail*, May 27, 2021.

48. Yasmeen Abutaleb and Josh Dawsey, "New Trump pandemic adviser pushes controversial 'herd immunity' strategy, worrying public health officials," *The Washington Post*, August 31, 2020.

49. Sharon LaFraniere, Katie Thomas, Noah Weiland, "Scientists Worry About Political Influence Over Coronavirus Vaccine Project," *The New York Times*, August 2, 2020.

50. Sabrina Siddiqui, "Biden Meets With Top Executives on Covid-19 Vaccine Mandate," *The Wall Street Journal*, September 15, 2021.

51. The Editorial Board, "Biden's Covid death milestone," *The Wall Street Journal*, November 25, 2021.

52. Jenny Strasburg and Laura Cooper, "Big Pharma Quietly Pushes Back on Global Tax Deal, Citing Covid-19 Role," *The Wall Street Journal*, July 27, 2021.

53. Jared S. Hopkins and Betsy McKay, "Merck Pill Intended to Treat Covid-19 Succeeds in Key Study," *The Wall Street Journal*, October 1, 2021.

54. Donald G. McNeil Jr., "With vaccines and a new administration, the pandemic will be tamed. But experts say the coming months "are going to be just horrible." *The New York Times*, November 30, 2020.

55. Michael Lewis, *The Premonition: A Pandemic Story*, W.W. Norton & Company, 2021, p. 299.

3. The Capitalists State

1. Edward Wong and Steve Lee Myers, "Officials push US-China relations toward point of no return," *The New York Times*, July 25, 2020.

2. Bill Powell, "How America's biggest companies made China great again," *Newsweek*, June 24, 2019.

3. Jeff Madrick, "Why the Working Class Votes Against Its Economic Interests," *The New York Times*, July 31, 2020.

4. Michael Powell, "Obama the Centrist Irks a Liberal Lion," *The New York Times*, January 7, 2011

5. Nicholas Carnes, "Which Millionaire Are You Voting For?" *The New York Times*, October 13, 2012.

6. Stephanie Condon, "Two Hundred Sixty-one Millionaires in Congress," CBSNews.com, November 17, 2010.

7. Karl Evers-Hillstrom, "Majority of lawmakers in 116th Congress are millionaires," opensecrets.org, April 23, 2020.

8. Chad Day, Luis Melgar and John McCormick, "Biden's Wealthiest Cabinet Officials: Zients, Lander, Rice Top the List," *The Wall Street Journal*, March 23, 2021.

9. Joseph Walker, "FDA nominee received industry fees," *The Wall Street Journal*, September 18, 2015.

10. Matthew Herper, "Robert Califf could transform the FDA—the right way," *Forbes*, September 16, 2015.

11. Ibid.

12. Liz Rappaport and Brody Mullions, "Goldman Turns Tables on Obama Campaign," *The Wall Street Journal*, October 9, 2012.

13. George Arnett, "Elitism in Britain. Breakdown by Profession," *The Guardian*, August 28, 2014.

14. Jonathan Wai and Kaja Perina, "Expertise in Journalism: Factors Shaping a Cognitive and Culturally Elite Profession," *The Journal of Expertise*, March, 2018.

15. Laurence H. Shoup, "The Council on Foreign Relations, the Biden Team, and Key Policy Outcomes," *Monthly Review*, May, 2021.

16. Julie Bykowicz and Tarini Parti, "Big Donors Spent Heavily on Failed Election Efforts," *The Wall Street Journal*, November 23, 2020.

17. Nicholas Confessore, Sarah Cohen, and Karen Yourish, "The Families Funding the 2016 Presidential Election," *The New York Times*, October 11, 2015.

18. Frank Bruni, "Hillary, Jeb and $$$$$$," *The New York Times*, February 21, 2015.

19. Gregory Zuckerman and Liz Hoffman, "Biden's Election Win Was a Big Bet for These Wall Street Executives," *The Wall Street Journal*, November 10, 2020.

20. Mike McIntire and Michael Luo, "White House Opens Door to Big Donors, and Lobbyists Slip In," *The New York Times*, April 14, 2012.

21. Kim Mackrael and Paul Vieira, "How Justin Trudeau Lost His Rock-Star Popularity," *The Wall Street Journal*, August 2, 2019.

22. Tim Kiladze, "Bay Street's hottest hires are former politicians: The latest, Navdeep Bains, is joining CIBC," *The Globe and Mail*, September 27, 2021.

23. Richard Harwood, "Ruling Class Journalists," *The Washington Post*, October 30, 1993.

24. Laurence H. Shoup, *Wall Street's Think Tank: The Council on Foreign Relations and the Empire of Neoliberal Geopolitics, 1976-2014*, Monthly Review Press, 2015; Laurence H. Shoup and William Minter, *Imperial Brain Trust: The Council on Foreign Relations and United States Foreign Policy*, Authors Choice Press, 2004.

25. Quoted in A.B. Abrams, *Immovable Object: North Korea's 70 Years at War with American Power*, Clarity Press, 2020, p. 401.

26. Eric Lipton and Brooke Williams, "Researchers or Corporate Allies? Think Tanks Blur the Line," *The New York Times*, August 7, 2016.

27. Eric Lipton, Nicholas Confessore and Brooke Williams, "Think Tank Scholar or Corporate Consultant? It Depends on the Day," *The New York Times*, August 8, 2016.

28. Eric Lipton, Nicholas Confessore and Brooke Williams, "Think Tank Scholar or Corporate Consultant? It Depends on the Day," *The New York Times*, August 8, 2016.

29. Damien Cave, "Australia Wilts from Climate Change. Why Can't Its Politicians Act?" *The New York Times*, August 21, 2018.

30. Amy Chozik, "Rupert Murdoch and President Trump: A Friendship of Convenience," *The New York Times*, December 23, 2017

31. Zaid Jilani, "When the world's richest billionaire owns your paper," FAIR, November 1, 2013.

32. Alan Cullison, "Ukraine's secret weapon: Feisty oligarch Ihor Kolomoisky", *The Wall Street Journal*, June 27, 2014.

33. Kate Murphy, Single-Payer & Interlocking Directorates: The corporate ties between insurance and media companies," *Extra!*, August, 2009.

34. Adam Johnson, "Top NYT Editor: 'We Are Pro-Capitalism, the Times Is in Favor of Capitalism'" FAIR, March 1, 2018.

35. Jonathan Wai and Kaja Perina, "Expertise in Journalism: Factors Shaping a Cognitive and Culturally Elite Profession," *The Journal of Expertise*, March, 2018.

36. Quoted in Peter Hart, "Syria's mobile weapons labs: Where have we heard this before?" *FAIR Blog*, December 20, 2012.

37. Tim Beal, "Korea and Imperialism," *The Palgrave Encyclopedia of Imperialism and Anti-Imperialism: Living Edition*, May 14, 2019, https://doi.org/10.1007/978-3-319-91206-6_92-1)

38. Radley Glasser and Steve Rendall, "For Media, 'Class War' Has Wealthy Victims: Rich getting richer seldom labeled as belligerents," *Extra!*, August, 2009.

39. "Tell Cable News: No More PR Pundits," FAIR Action Alert, February 17, 2010.

40. Cited in Donald Gutstein, *Not a Conspiracy Theory: How Business Propaganda Hijacks Democracy*, Key Porter Books, 2009, p.306.

41. Robert Reich, "Why the major media marginalize Bernie," March 30, 2016, http://robertreich.org/post/141981929755 .

42. Marc Fisher, "The covid endgame: Is the pandemic over already? Or are there years to go?" *The Washington Post*, September 4, 2021.

4. The Capitalists' Nanny State

1. Linsey McGoey, *No Such Thing as a Free Gift: The Gates Foundation and the Price of Philanthropy*, Verso, 2015, p. 83.

2. Joseph E. Stiglitz, Todd N. Tucker, and Gabriel Zucman, "Why Capitalism's Salvation Depends on Taxation," *Foreign Affairs*, January/February 2020.

3. Quoted in Hans Schmidt, *Maverick Marine: General Smedley D. Butler and the Contradictions of American Military History*, Lexington: University Press of Kentucky, 1998, p. 231.

4. Quoted in "Notes from the Editors," *Monthly Review*, July, 1999.

5. Arno J. Mayer, "Untimely reflections upon the state of the world," *Counterpunch.org*, January 16, 2015.

6. A.B. Abrams, *Power and Primacy: A Recent History of Western Intervention in the Asia-Pacific*, Peter Lang, 2019, p. 617.

7. "Is China ramping up military spending?" *Xinhua*, March 09, 2021.

8. "After the Trade War, a Real War with China?" Remarks to the St. Petersburg Conference on World Affairs Ambassador Chas W. Freeman, Jr. (USFS, Ret.), 12 February 2019.

9. Thomas Grove, "The New Iron Curtain: Russian Missile Defense Challenges US Air Power," *The Wall Street Journal*, January 23, 2019.

10. Yaroslav Trofimov, "Is Europe Ready to Defend Itself?" *The Wall Street Journal*, January 4, 2019.

11. Cheong Wook-Sik, "The arms race lining the military-industrial complex's pockets," *The Hankyoreh*, October 16, 2021.

12. Cheong Wook-Sik, "The arms race lining the military-industrial complex's pockets," *The Hankyoreh*, October 16, 2021.

13. Robert Fisk, "9/11 remembered: Robert Fisk's close encounter with Osama bin Laden, the man who shook the world," *The Independent*, September 11, 2018.

14. Robert A. Pape, *Dying to Win: The Strategic Logic of Suicide Terrorism*, Random House, 2006, p. 124.

15. Robert Fisk, "9/11 remembered: Robert Fisk's close encounter with Osama bin Laden, the man who shook the world," *The Independent*, September 11, 2018.

16. Robert A. Pape, *Dying to Win: The Strategic Logic of Suicide Terrorism*, Random House, 2006, p. 114.

17. Ibid, p. 118.

18. Ibid, p. 118.

19. Ibid, p. 118.

20. Karl Marx, "The Indian Revolt," *The New York Daily Tribune*, September 16, 1857.

21. Arnaud Borchgrave, "Text of UPI interview with Haig," UPI, January 7, 2002.

22. William Appleman Williams, *The Tragedy of American Diplomacy*, W.W. Norton & Company, 2009, p. 72.

23. Ibid, p. 84.

24. David Vine, *The United States of War: A Global History of America's Endless Conflicts, from Columbus to the Islamic State*, University of California Press, 2021, p. xiv.

25. David Vine, *The United States of War: A Global History of America's Endless Conflicts, from Columbus to the Islamic State*, University of California Press, 2021, p. xv.

26. William Appleman Williams, *The Great Evasion*, Quadrangle Books, 1964, p. 74-75.

27. James T. Areddy, "China's Industrial Planning Evolves, Stirring U.S. Concerns," *The Wall Street Journal*, September 5, 2021.

28. Fred Block and Matthew R Keller, "Where do innovations come from? Transformations in the U.S. national innovation system, 1970-2006," Technology and Innovation Foundation, July 2008. http://www.itif.org/files/Where_do_innovations_come_from.pdf.

29. Seumas Milne, "Budget 2012: George Osborne is stuck in a failed economic model, circa 1979," *The Guardian*, March 20, 2012.

30. Mariana Mazzucato, "Capitalism After the Pandemic: Getting the Recovery Right," *Foreign Affairs*, October 2, 2020.

31. Israel Meléndez Ayala and Alicia Kennedy, "How the U.S. Dictates What Puerto Rico Eats," *The New York Times*, October 1, 2021.

32. Stu Woo and Drew Hinshaw, "U.S. Fight Against Chinese 5G Efforts Shifts From Threats to Incentives," *The Wall Street Journal*, June 14, 2021.

33. Alexandra Wexler and Stu Woo, "U.S. Fund Set Up to Counter China's Influence Backs Covid-19 Vaccine Maker in Africa," *The Wall Street Journal*, June 30, 2021.

34. Stu Woo and Drew Hinshaw, "U.S. Fight Against Chinese 5G Efforts Shifts From Threats to Incentives," *The Wall Street Journal*, June 14, 2021.

35. Editorial Board, "Huawei and the U.S.-China Tech War," *The Wall Street Journal*, June 9, 2020.

36. Dan Strumpf, "US Set Out to Hobble China's Huawei, and So It Has," *The Wall Street Journal*, October 7, 2021.

37. Editorial Board, "Huawei and the U.S.-China Tech War," *The Wall Street Journal*, June 9, 2020.

38. William Mauldin and Chao Deng, "US-China talks stuck in rut over Huawei," *The Wall Street Journal*, July 17, 2019.

39. Yuka Hayashi, "U.S., Europe Team Up to Address Chip Shortage, Tech Issues," *The Wall Street Journal*, September 29, 2021.

40. Josh Zumbrun and Daniel Michaels, "Boeing Subsidies Merit EU Tariffs on $4 Billion in U.S. Goods, WTO Rules," *The Wall Street Journal*, October 13, 2020.

41. David E. Sanger, Catie Edmondson, David McCabe and Thomas Kaplan, "Senate Poised to Pass Huge Industrial Policy Bill to Counter China," *The New York Times*, June 7, 2021.

42. David E. Sanger, Catie Edmondson, David McCabe and Thomas Kaplan, "Senate Poised to Pass Huge Industrial Policy Bill to Counter China," *The New York Times*, June 7, 2021.

43. Gerald F. Seib, "In Biden World, Economic Policy Is National Security Policy," *The Wall Street Journal*, February 15, 2021.

44. Austen Hufford and Bob Tita, "Manufacturers Want Biden to Boost 'Buy American' Practices," *The Wall Street Journal*, January 3, 2021.

45. Gerald F. Seib, "The Really Critical Infrastructure Need: American-Made Semiconductors," *The Wall Street Journal*, July 26, 2021.

46. John D. McKinnon, "China Rivalry Spurs Republicans and Democrats to Align on Tech Spending," *The Wall Street Journal* April 14, 2021.

47. Jacob M. Schlesinger, "Biden's Economic Plan Would Redistribute Trillions and Expand Government," *The Wall Street Journal*, April 29, 2021.

48. Neil Irwin, "The Pandemic Is Showing Us How Capitalism Is Amazing, and Inadequate," *The New York Times*, November 14, 2020.

49. David E. Sanger, Catie Edmondson, David McCabe and Thomas Kaplan, "Senate Poised to Pass Huge Industrial Policy Bill to Counter China," *The New York Times*, June 7, 2021.

50. "Barack Obama's State of the Union address – full text," *The Guardian*, January 26, 2011.

51. Andrew Browne, "China's dream is Apple's nightmare: US tech firms cave for Beijing's rules," *The Wall Street Journal*, August 8, 2017.

5. Capitalist Pharmacy
1. N. Bukharin and E. Preobrazhensky, *The ABC of Communism*, Penguin Books, 1970, p. 88.
2. Sharon Lerner, "Merck sells federally financed Covid pill to US for 40 times what it costs to make," *The Intercept*, October 5, 2021.
3. Betsy McKay and Jared S. Hopkins, "Behind a new pill to treat Covid: A husband and wife team and a hunch," *The Wall Street Journal*, December 20, 2021.
4. Sharon Lerner, "Merck sells federally financed Covid pill to US for 40 times what it costs to make," *The Intercept*, October 5, 2021.
5. Emily Bobrow, "Vaccine Expert Paul Offit Believes Science Will Win in the End," *The Wall Street Journal*, February 5, 2021.
6. "The people's prescription: Reimagining health innovation to deliver public value," UCL Institute for Innovation and Public Purpose, October, 2018.
7. Donald G. McNeil Jr., "Gates Offers Grim Global Health Report, and Some Optimism," *The New York Times*, September 14, 2020.
8. John M. Barry, *The Great Influenza: The Story of the Deadliest Pandemic in History*, Penguin Books, 2018, pp. 453-454.
9. Kim Tingley, "We're Getting Close to 'Universal' Vaccines. It Hasn't Been Easy," *The New York Times*, December 8, 2021.
10. "Mike Davis on pandemics, super-capitalism and the struggles of tomorrow," *MRZine*, April 7, 2020.
11. Equivalent to the number of deaths during the Great Influenza of 1918 to 1920, adjusted to today's population.
12. Maryn McKenna, "The antibiotic paradox: why companies can't afford to create life-saving drugs," *Nature* 584, 338-341, 2020.
13. Mariana Mazucatto et al., The people's prescription: Re-imagining health innovation to deliver public value, Institute for Innovation and Public Purpose, October, 2018.
14. Gabriele Steinhauser and Denise Roland, "World's First Malaria Vaccine Gets WHO Backing," *The Wall Street Journal*, October 6, 2021.
15. Morris Pearl and William Lazonick, "With working Americans' survival at stake, the US is bailing out the richest," *The Guardian*, April 13, 2020.
16. Morris Pearl and William Lazonick, "With working Americans' survival at stake, the US is bailing out the richest," *The Guardian*, April 13, 2020.
17. Mariana Mazucatto et al., The people's prescription: Re-imagining health innovation to deliver public value, Institute for Innovation and Public Purpose, October, 2018.
18. Pam Belluck, Sheila Kaplan and Rebecca Robbins, "How an Unproven Alzheimer's Drug Got Approved," *The New York Times*, July 19, 2021.
19. Ibid.
20. Pam Belluck and Rebecca Robbins, "F.D.A. Approves Alzheimer's Drug Despite Fierce Debate Over Whether It Works," *The New York Times*, June 7, 2021.
21. Pam Belluck, "Biogen slashes price of Alzheimer's drug Aduhelm, as it faces obstacles," *The New York Times*, December 20, 2021.

22. Joseph Walker, "Biogen's New Alzheimer's Drug Beyond Research for Many Patients," *The Wall Street Journal*, August 27, 2021.

23. Betsy McKay and Jared S. Hopkins, "Behind a new pill to treat Covid: A husband and wife team and a hunch," *The Wall Street Journal*, December 20, 2021.

24. Carolyn Y. Johnson and Katie Shepherd, "FDA advisers narrowly recommend authorization of first antiviral pill to treat covid-19," *The Washington Post*, November 30, 2021.

25. Jared S. Hopkins and Betsy McKay, "Merck's Covid-19 Pill Backed by FDA Advisers," *The Wall Street Journal*, November 30, 2021.

26. Carolyn Y. Johnson and Katie Shepherd, "FDA advisers narrowly recommend authorization of first antiviral pill to treat covid-19," *The Washington Post*, November 30, 2021.

27. Sharon Lerner, "Merck sells federally financed Covid pill to US for 40 times what it costs to make," *The Intercept*, October 5, 2021.

28. Joseph Walker, "Biogen's New Alzheimer's Drug Beyond Research for Many Patients," *The Wall Street Journal*, August 27, 2021.

29. Mariana Mazucatto et al., The people's prescription: Re-imagining health innovation to deliver public value, Institute for Innovation and Public Purpose, October, 2018.

30. Karen Attiah, "The Biden administration needs to share the Moderna vaccine recipe with the world now," *The Washington Post*, October 18, 2021.

6. The Billionaire

1. Bertolt Brecht, A Worker Reads History.

2. Paraphrasing Teju Cole. The white savior supports brutal policies in the morning, founds charities in the afternoon, and receives awards in the evening.—Teju Cole, Twitter, March 8, 2012.

3. Linsey McGoey, *No Such Thing as a Free Gift: The Gates Foundation and the Price of Philanthropy*, Verso, 2015, p. 176.

4. Norman Bethune, "Take the Private Profit Out of Medicine," April 17, 1936, in Roderick Stewart (Ed.), *The Mind of Norman Bethune*, Fitzhenry and Whiteside, 2002, pp. 46-53.

5. Jeremy Loffredo and Michele Greenstein, "Why the Bill Gates global health empire promises more empire and less public health," *The Grayzone*, July 8, 2020.

6. Megan Twohey and Nicholas Kulish, "Bill Gates, the Virus and the Quest to Vaccinate the World," *The New York Times*, November 23, 2020.

7. Tim Schwab, "While the Poor Get Sick, Bill Gates Just Gets Richer," *The Nation*, October 5, 2020.

8. Ibid.

9. Michele Greenstein and Jeremy Loffredo, "Why the Bill Gates global health empire promises more empire and less public health," *The Grayzone*, July 8, 2020.

10. Megan Twohey and Nicholas Kulish, "Bill Gates, the Virus and the Quest to Vaccinate the World," *The New York Times*, November 23, 2020.

11 Laurie Garrett, "Money or Die: A Watershed Moment for Global Public Health," *Foreign Affairs*, March 6, 2012.

12. Nina Burleigh, *Virus: Vaccinations, the CDC, and the Hijacking of America's Response to the Pandemic*, Seven Stories Press, 2021, p. 22.

13. Frank W. Snowden, *Epidemics and Society: From the Black Death to the Present*, Yale University Press, 2020, p. 364.

14. Ibid, p. 375.

15. Ibid, p. 365.

16. Gabriele Steinhauser and Denise Roland, "World's First Malaria Vaccine Gets WHO Backing," *The Wall Street Journal*, October 6, 2021.

17. Megan Twohey and Nicholas Kulish, "Bill Gates, the Virus and the Quest to Vaccinate the World," *The New York Times*, November 23, 2020.

18. Linsey McGoey, *No Such Thing as a Free Gift: The Gates Foundation and the Price of Philanthropy*, Verso, 2015, p. 244.

19. Tim Schwab, "Bill Gates's Charity Paradox," *The Nation*, March 17, 2020.

20. Ruchir Sharma, "The billionaire boom: how the super rich soaked up Covid cash," *The Financial Times*, May 14, 2021.

21. Tim Schwab, "Bill Gates's Charity Paradox," *The Nation*, March 17, 2020.

22. Ibid.

23. Megan Twohey and Nicholas Kulish, "Bill Gates, the Virus and the Quest to Vaccinate the World," *The New York Times*, November 23, 2020.

24. Ed Augustin and Natalie Kitroeff, "Coronavirus Vaccine Nears Final Tests in Cuba. Tourists May Be Inoculated," *The Wall Street Journal*, February 17, 2021.

25. Peter S. Goodman, Apoorva Mandavilli, Rebecca Robbins and Matina Stevis-Gridneff, "What Would It Take to Vaccinate the World Against Covid?" *The New York Times*, May 15, 2021.

26. Peter Loftus, "Who invented Covid-19 vaccines? Drugmakers battle over patents," *The Wall Street Journal*, December 29, 2021.

27. Michael Lewis, *The Premonition: A Pandemic Story*, W.W. Norton & Company, 2021, p. 178.

28. Ilari Kaila and Joona-Hermanni Makinen, "Finland Had a Patent-Free COVID-19 Vaccine Nine Months Ago—But Still Went With Big Pharma," *Jacobin*, February 28, 2021.

29. "'Government Money That's Gone into Vaccine Development Is Being Privatized by a Handful of Companies': CounterSpin interview with James Love on Bill Gates & vaccine politics," FAIR, May 12, 2021.

30. Alan Macleod, "Documents show Bill Gates has given $319 million to media outlets to promote his global agenda," *The Grayzone*, November 21, 2021.

31. Robert B. Reich, "Why Philanthropy Actually Hurts Rather Than Helps Some of the World's Worst Problems, George Joseph," *In These Times*, December 28, 2015.

32. Sheryl Gay Stolberg and Rebecca Robbins, "Moderna and U.S. at Odds Over Vaccine Patent Rights," *The New York Times*, November 9, 2021.

33. Bill Gates, "Bill Gates: Here's how to make up for lost time on covid-19," *The Washington Post*, March 31, 2020.

34. Scott W. Atlas, "A Pandemic of Misinformation," *The Wall Street Journal*, December 21, 2020.

35. Nina Burleigh, *Virus: Vaccinations, the CDC, and the Hijacking of America's Response to the Pandemic*, Seven Stories Press. 2021. p. 107.

36. Selam Gebrekidan and Matt Apuzzo, "Rich Countries Signed Away a Chance to Vaccinate the World," *The Wall Street Journal*, March 21, 2021.

37. Sharon LaFraniere, Katie Thomas, Noah Weiland, David Gelles, Sheryl Gay Stolberg and Denise Grady, "Politics, Science and the Remarkable Race for a Coronavirus Vaccine," *The New York Times*, November 21, 2020.

38. Sheryl Gay Stolberg and Rebecca Robbins, "Moderna and U.S. at Odds Over Vaccine Patent Rights" *The New York Times*, November 9, 2021.

39. Dan Diamond, "Moderna halts patent fight over coronavirus vaccine with federal government," *The Washington Post*, December 17, 2021.

7. The Henchman

1. N. Bukharin and E. Preobrazhensky, *The ABC of Communism*, Penguin Books, 1970, p. 422.

2. William Haseltine, "We're wasting time talking about herd immunity," CNN, July 13, 2020.

3. "Scientific consensus on the COVID-19 pandemic: we need to act now," *The Lancet*, October 15, 2020.

4. Jennifer Abbasi, "Anthony Fauci, MD, on COVID-19 Vaccines, Schools, and Larry Kramer," *The Journal of the American Medical Association*, June 8, 2020.

5. Ibid.

6. David E. Sanger, David D. Kirkpatrick, Carl Zimmer, Katie Thomas and Sui-Lee Wee, "Profits and Pride at Stake, the Race for a Vaccine Intensifies," *The New York Times*, May 2, 2020.

7. Lauren Webber, "A Top Immunologist on Why Coronavirus Is Killing More African-Americans," *The Wall Street Journal*, April 22, 2020.

8. Carl Zimmer, Knvul Sheikh and Noah Weiland, "A New Entry in the Race for a Coronavirus Vaccine: Hope," *The New York Times*, May 20, 2020.

9. Stuart A. Thompson, "How Long Will a Vaccine Really Take?" *The New York Times*, April 30, 2020.

10. Jared S. Hopkins and Jonathan D. Rockoff, "Race for Coronavirus Vaccine Accelerates as Pfizer Says U.S. Testing to Begin Next Week," *The Wall Street Journal*, April 28, 2020.

11. David E. Sanger, David D. Kirkpatrick, Carl Zimmer, Katie Thomas and Sui-Lee Wee, "Profits and Pride at Stake, the Race for a Vaccine Intensifies," *The New York Times*, May 2, 2020.

12. Ibid.

13. Jared S. Hopkins and Jonathan D. Rockoff, "Race for Coronavirus Vaccine Accelerates as Pfizer Says U.S. Testing to Begin Next Week," *The Wall Street Journal*, April 28, 2020.

14. Jan Hoffman, "Mistrust of a Coronavirus Vaccine Could Imperil Widespread Immunity," *The New York Times*, July 18, 2020.

15. "Why were US media silent on Pfizer vaccine deaths?: Global Times editorial," *Global Times*, January 18, 2021.

16. Paul A. Offit, *You Bet Your Life: From Blood Transfusions to Mass Vaccination, the Long and Risky History of Medical Innovations*, Basic Books, 2021, p. 8.

17. Ibid, p. 209.

18. Peter Loftus and Susan Pulliam, "People Harmed by Coronavirus Vaccines Will Have Little Recourse," *The Wall Street Journal*, October 11, 2020.

19. Noel Weiland and David E. Sanger, "Trump Administration Selects Five Coronavirus Vaccine Candidates as Finalists," *The New York Times,* June 3, 2020.
20. Jeremy Loffredo and Michele Greenstein, "Why the Bill Gates global health empire promises more empire and less public health," *The Grayzone,* July 8, 2020.
21. "Evaluating covid-19 vaccine efficacy and safety in the post-authorisation phase," *The British Medical Journal,* 23 December 2021. https://doi.org/10.1136/bmj-2021-067570.
22. Ibid.
23. Ibid.
24. Ibid.
25. Marc Siegel, "Is Moderna the Tortoise in the Vaccine Race?" *The Wall Street Journal,* September 6, 2021.
26. Gretchen Vogel, "The COVID-19 vaccine booster debate intensifies," *Science,* August 27, 2021.
27. David E. Sanger, David D. Kirkpatrick, Carl Zimmer, Katie Thomas and Sui-Lee Wee, "Profits and Pride at Stake, the Race for a Vaccine Intensifies," *The New York Times,* May 2, 2020.
28. Robert M. Kaplan, "A False Narrative About 'Misinformation' and Covid Vaccines," *The Wall Street Journal,* August 3, 2021.
29. Sarah Toy, "Why Some Healthcare Workers Would Rather Lose Their Jobs Than Get Vaccinated," *The New York Times,* October 22, 2021.
30. Linsey McGoey, *No Such Thing as a Free Gift: The Gates Foundation and the Price of Philanthropy,* Verso, 2015, p 104-105.
31. Ibid, p 103-104.
32. Ibid, p. 161.
33. Lee Fang, "Pfizer is lobbying to thwart whistleblowers from exposing corporate fraud," *The Intercept,* November 29, 2021.
34. Laura Spinney, "Drugs, money and misleading evidence," Nature, June 29, 2020.
35. Jon Jereidini and Leemon B. McHenry, *The Illusion of Evidence-Based Medicine: Exposing the Crisis of Credibility in Clinical Research,* Wakefield Press, 2020.
36. Nina Burleigh, *Virus: Vaccinations, the CDC, and the Hijacking of America's Response to the Pandemic,* Seven Stories Press. 2021. p. 26.
37. Victor F. Zonana, "Why we shouldn't over-promise on vaccines," *The Washington Post,* September 1, 2020.
38. Howard P. Segal, "Practical Utopias: America as Techno-Fix Nation," Utopian Studies, Vol. 28, No. 2 (2017), pp. 231-246.
39. Jill Lepore, "Elon Musk is building a sci-fi world and the rest of us are trapped in it." *The New York Times,* November 4, 2021.
40. Sabrina Siddiqui, "Biden Meets With Top Executives on Covid-19 Vaccine Mandate," *The Wall Street Journal,* September 15, 2021.
41. Yasmeen Abutaleb and Josh Dawsey, "Trump's soft touch with China's Xi worries advisers who say more is needed to combat coronavirus outbreak," *The Washington Post,* February 16, 2020.
42. Nina Burleigh, *Virus: Vaccinations, the CDC, and the Hijacking of America's Response to the Pandemic,* Seven Stories Press. 2021. p. 115.
43. Sheryl Gay Stolberg, "Trump and Friends Got Coronavirus Care Many Others Couldn't," *The New York Times,* December 9, 2020.

44. Nina Burleigh, *Virus: Vaccinations, the CDC, and the Hijacking of America's Response to the Pandemic,* Seven Stories Press, 2021, p. 34.

45. Ibid, p. 43.

46. Ibid, p. 48-49.

47. Kat Eschner, "New Books That Look at the Pandemic and Its Consequences," *The New York Times,* August 12, 2021.

48. Ryan Dube and Luciana Magalhaes, "For Covid-19 Vaccines, Latin America Turns to China and Russia," *The Wall Street Journal,* February. 24, 2021.

49. Ibid.

50. The Editorial Board, "For Ontario, a few small steps today can prevent a big fourth pandemic wave tomorrow," *The Globe and Mail,* November 9, 2021.

51. The Editorial Board, "Biden's twin crises of the pandemic demand action, not anger," *The Globe and Mail,* December 20, 2021.

52. Benjamin Mueller, "U.K. and U.S. Officials Spar Over 'Vaccine Nationalism'," *The New York Times,* December 3, 2020.

53. David Cole and Daniel Mach, "We Work at the A.C.L.U. Here's What We Think About Vaccine Mandates." *The New York Times,* September 2, 2021.

54. Donald G. McNeil Jr., "With vaccines and a new administration, the pandemic will be tamed. But experts say the coming months "are going to be just horrible." *The New York Times,* November 30, 2020.

55. Krishna Pokharel and Eric Bellman, "With Covid-19 Pandemic Dragging On, Some Countries Say They Can't Afford to Fight," *The Wall Street Journal,* November 20, 2020.

56. Norimitu Onishi, Constant Mehuet, and Leontine Gallois, "Omicron strains France's social contract on Covid," *The New York Times,* December 31, 2021.

57. Jenny Strasburg and Laura Cooper, "Big Pharma Quietly Pushes Back on Global Tax Deal, Citing Covid-19 Role," *The Wall Street Journal,* July 27, 2021.

58. Krishna Pokharel and Eric Bellman, "With Covid-19 Pandemic Dragging On, Some Countries Say They Can't Afford to Fight," *The Wall Street Journal,* November 20, 2020.

59. Annabelle Timsit, "Health experts want Britain to bring back covid restrictions. The government says: 'We don't want to go back," *The Washington Post,* October 20, 2021.

60. Natasha Khan, "China Sticks to Covid-Zero Policies, Despite Rising Pressure to Ease Restrictions," *The Wall Street Journal,* October 28, 2021; Liyan Qi and Natasha Khan, "Covid-19 Lockdowns Ripple Across China—'I Wonder How Long I Can Hang On'," *The Wall Street Journal,* November 4, 2021.

61. Liyan Qi, "China's Covid-19 lockdowns starting to sting," *The Wall Street Journal,* December 15, 2021.

62. Stephanie Nolen, "Here's Why Developing Countries Can Make mRNA Covid Vaccines, *The New York Times,* October 22, 2021.

63. Jared S. Hopkins and Matt Grossman, "Pfizer Raises Covid-19 Vaccine Forecast as Sales More Than Double," *The Wall Street Journal,* November 2, 2021.

64. Annie Linskey, Yasmeen Abutaleb and Tyler Pager, "Four weeks in July: Inside the Biden administration's struggle to contain the delta surge," *The Washington Post,* August 21, 2021.

65. Jared S. Hopkins, "Annual Covid-19 Vaccine Booster Shots Likely Needed, Pfizer CEO Says," *The Wall Street Journal*, April 15, 2021.

66. Sharon LaFraniere, "Biden Administration Plans for Vaccine Boosters, Perhaps by Fall," *The New York Times*, August 14, 2021.

67. Apoorva Mandavilli, "Vaccine Effectiveness Against Infection May Wane, C.D.C. Studies Find," *The New York Times*, August 18, 2021.

68. Carl Zimmer and Sharon LaFraniere, "Moderna says its vaccine's protection holds through six months," *The Wall Street Journal*, August 5, 2021.

69. WHO Director-General's opening remarks at the media briefing on Covid-19, 22 December 2021.

70. Joseph Walker, "Pfizer to Ask Regulators to Authorize Covid-19 Vaccine Booster," *The Wall Street Journal*, July 8, 2021.

71. Sharon LaFraniere and Noah Weiland, "Scale Back Booster Plan for Now," *The New York Times*, September 3, 2021.

72. Noah Weiland and Sharon LaFraniere, "Two Top F.D.A. Vaccine Regulators Are Set to Depart During a Crucial Period," *The New York Times*, August 31, 2021.

73. Philip R. Krause and Lucian Borio, "The Biden administration has been sidelining vaccine experts," *The Washington Post*, December 16, 2021.

74. Sarah Toy, "Covid-19 Boosters Aren't Necessary Yet, Group of Scientists Say," *The Wall Street Journal*, September 13, 2021.

75. Sharon LaFraniere and Noah Weiland, "F.D.A. Panel Recommends Booster for Many Moderna Vaccine Recipients," *The New York Times*, October 14, 2021.

76. Noah Weiland and Sharon LaFraniere, "F.D.A. Authorizes Moderna and Johnson & Johnson Booster Shots," *The New York Times*, October 20, 2021.

77. Sharon LaFraniere, Noah Weiland and Carl Zimmer, "F.D.A. Panel Unanimously Recommends Johnson & Johnson Booster Shots," *The New York Times*, October 15, 2021.

78. WHO Director-General's opening remarks at the media briefing on Covid-19, 14 December 2021.

79. Ibid.

80. Ibid.

81. Chip Cutter, Douglas Belkin, and Ruth Simon, "Nation's January goal: Stay open, despite Omicron," *The Wall Street Journal*, December 22, 2021.

82. Lee Fang, "Biden's inner circle maintains close ties to vaccine makers, disclosures reveal," *The Intercept*, March 24, 2021.

Conclusion

1. N. Bukharin and E. Preobrazhensky, *The ABC of Communism*, Penguin Books, 1970, p. 82.

2. Peter Loftus, "Who invented Covid-19 vaccines? Drugmakers battle over patents," *The Wall Street Journal*, December 29, 2021.

3. Remarks by Vice President Harris on the Indo-Pacific Region, White House, August 24, 2021, Gardens by the Bay, Singapore, Singapore.

4. Joseph R. Biden, "Why America Must Lead Again," *Foreign Affairs*, March/April 2020.

5. Ed Cara, "The World Just Hit 5 Million Official Covid-19 Deaths, but the Real Toll Is Much Worse," *Gizmodo*, October 29, 2021.

INDEX*

* Page references in **bold** indicate a table.

Printed by Imprimerie Gauvin
Gatineau, Québec